PRAISE FOR TRACEY COX
AND *GREAT SEX STARTS AT 50*

"Frank, forthright, and at times hysterically funny."

—*Cosmopolitan UK*

"Cox is fantastically unshockable. She has the practical, unsqueamish air of a doctor without the white coat."

—*The Observer*

"What distinguishes her from other so-called sexperts is an ability to talk with candor and a sense of empathy.... This is the heart of her appeal, the ability to talk about sex in a universal way."

—*The London Times*

"Tracey Cox is stunningly well informed about sex. She can tell a G-spot from an A-spot and could probably find both of them before the rest of us have got the map references."

—*The Mirror*

"*Great Sex Starts at 50* is perhaps Tracey Cox's most intimate book to date. After 20 years answering sex questions from people all over the world, she knows the questions everyone is wondering about ("Is something wrong with my libido, or am I just bored?") and answers them all with her trademark sanity and compassion. Hoping to keep having great sex for the rest of your life? Be sure to keep this book next to your bed."

—Stephen Snyder, MD, author of *Love Worth Making: How to Have Ridiculously Great Sex in a Long-Lasting Relationship*

GREAT
SEX
— STARTS AT —
50

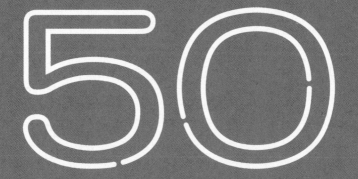

Age-Proof Your Libido
& Transform Your Sex Life

TRACEY COX

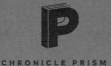

CHRONICLE PRISM

First published in North America in 2021 by
Chronicle Books LLC.
Originally published in the United Kingdom in 2019 by Murdoch Books.

This book is written as a source of information only. The information
contained in this book should by no means be considered a substitute for the
advice of a qualified medical professional, who should always be consulted
before beginning any new exercise or other health program.

Library of Congress Cataloging-in-Publication Data available.

ISBN 978-1-7972-0788-9

Manufactured in the United States of America.

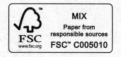

Author photograph © John Scott.
Design by Laura Palese.
Typesetting by Maureen Forys, Happenstance Type-O-Rama.
Typeset in Freight Text, Omnes, Mohr, Bryant, and Veneer Clean.

10 9 8 7 6 5 4 3 2 1

Chronicle books and gifts are available at special quantity
discounts to corporations, professional associations, literacy programs,
and other organizations. For details and discount information, please contact
our premiums department at corporatesales@chroniclebooks.com
or at 1-800-759-0190.

CHRONICLE PRISM

Chronicle Prism is an imprint of Chronicle Books LLC,
680 Second Street, San Francisco, California 94107

www.chronicleprism.com

TO MY HUSBAND, MILES,
MY EVERYTHING

CONTENTS

GET READY FOR THE
RIDE OF YOUR LIFE!

ASKED TO CONJURE UP AN image of a middle-aged woman 20 years ago, most would picture a permed, stout female in sensible shoes, puttering about in the garden. Look up Jennifer Lopez—who recently turned 50—and you'll see things have changed. My God, have they changed! Fifty-plus looks nothing like it used to. We have powerful female role models other generations never had: ageless beauties like Helen Mirren, the vivacious Taraji P. Henson, nutty old Madonna still wearing her fishnets, Christine Lagarde, Annie Leibovitz, Annie Lennox, Isabelle Huppert, Jennifer Doudna, and Michelle Obama. None of these women got the memo that you're meant to become sexless, invisible, and dull when you hit half a century. We're different from our mothers when it comes to sex, as well. We're better educated than ever before. We're aware of the benefits of testosterone supplements and know that Hormone Replacement Therapy (HRT) can keep our sex organs in good condition, as well as our moods stable. We exercise more, do yoga and Pilates, eat better, feel and dress younger.

As a society, we're much more open about things like menopause, and—love it or loathe it—there is absolutely no doubt that *Fifty Shades of Grey* had a massive impact on middle-aged women, reminding us of how good sex used to be when it was interesting rather than routine and repetitive. Your kids might look disgusted at the thought that you're still at it, but some older women are having more sex, and more satisfying sex, than ever before.

And yet . . . if it were all plain sailing, there would be no reason for me to write this book, would there? Something happens to us sexually at 50. Our desire for sex plummets. Low desire is the most common sex issue affecting older people—and it's twice as common in women. Lots of couples don't talk about dwindling desire, where any type of physical intimacy starts to feel awkward and, without acknowledgment, all affection stops and couples drift apart. There are a lot of older people flatlining and free-falling toward a sexless future—and panicking about it.

It's not that we're all just lazy, either. Even if 50 is the new 35, our bodies are still changing. Menopause brings with it a whole set of challenges, from painful sex and dry vaginas to bottomed-out libidos and body-image issues. Meanwhile, many men worry about penises that don't perform like they used to, suffering a crisis of confidence as they grapple with erectile dysfunction and the mixed blessing that is Viagra. Toss in such pedestrian aging realities as knee pain, stiff backs, arthritis, and unwanted sexual side effects from common post-50 medications, and sex can become a source of stress rather than pleasure.

Other challenges go beyond the physical: is it possible to reignite desire after decades with the same person? What do you do when you love your partner desperately but no longer want to have sex with them? Is it possible to have a healthy relationship if there is no sex? And how do you cope with the mess that's left when infidelity visits? Happily, information and enthusiasm are all it takes to work through a lot of these issues and reclaim a robust sex life. Why bother? Sex isn't just for fun; it keeps us healthy as well. It's great for the immune system, our hearts, and muscle strength. One study found the death rate halved for middle-aged men who reported the highest number of orgasms. Research also shows that sex helps to reduce blood pressure, lower stress, lift our mood, and even improve our memory. Regular orgasms are crucial for both our emotional and physical well-being; they help us sleep, make us feel more relaxed, and release endorphins that make us feel lighthearted. It's undeniable: there's a strong correlation between sexual intimacy and a sense of well-being for people of all ages.

This book isn't about trying to stay young—either in attitude or physicality. It's not about desperately trying to turn back the clock. It's about empowering you with information and practical solutions so you can be the best version of yourself, able to enjoy your relationships, whatever situation you're in, inspired and ready to live the second half of your life as happily as the first.

We are all unique, and I've written this book with all of you in mind, whether you're in a long-term relationship, newly single, happily settled for life, or somewhere in between. It's for everyone on the sexuality spectrum—straight, bisexual, lesbians, women who love sex, women who dread sex, and women who've never quite gotten what all the fuss was about. Most of all, it's for women who once loved sex but have lost enthusiasm due to the aging process. I've aimed this book at women, but it's designed to be shared with your partner—male or female—so both of you can benefit.

I interviewed hundreds of women aged 45 to 80 for this book, and their stories both uplifted me and broke my heart. Some are having great sex; others have decided not to have sex at all. One woman had her first orgasm at 45; another had hers at 17 and continues to have them, with the same person, in her seventies. There's something to be learned from all of these women, and you'll find their case histories and quotes scattered throughout the book.

I'm 59 and this is my 17th book on sex and relationships. My first was *Hot Sex: How to Do It*, published 20 years ago. Maybe you read it and have gotten older with me. It became one of the best-selling books of its time, selling over one million copies worldwide and translated into more than 20 languages. *Hot Sex* was one of the first sex books to offer practical, step-by-step advice that was tried and tested and nonjudgmental. It tells you everything you need to know to have great sex . . . under the age of 50. Until you hit 50 yourself, you have no idea that sex is a totally different ball game in the second half-century.

This is the grown-up's version of *Hot Sex*. I hope you find it real, reassuring, honest, and (hopefully) funny. Most of all, I hope you find it useful—a book you can dip into and out of, that's there by your side from now on. Kind of like a best friend who's super-knowledgeable about sex. If I really wanted to flatter myself, I'd imagine you giving it to your daughters, friends, and workmates when they hit their fifties. I hope you enjoy reading it as much as I loved writing it.

SIX TRUTHS ABOUT SEX THAT WILL NEVER CHANGE

1. One of the most powerful aphrodisiacs is being desired. Knowing someone really wants you beats even outstanding sexual technique any day.

2. The most erotic sex of your life won't necessarily include an orgasm. When you're totally immersed in the experience, having an orgasm becomes irrelevant. This is why orgasm-focused sex misses the point entirely.

3. Saying no to sex now and then is no bad thing. It means you feel comfortable saying no, leaving your partner reassured that when you say yes, you are really in the mood for it.

4. Sex is psychophysiological. This means you have to keep your brain stimulated for your genitals to sit up and pay attention.

5. Sex isn't something that "comes naturally." We aren't born knowing how to make love to someone. It's something we learn.

6. True arousal is much more than feeling "wet" or "hard." You feel it in the whole of your body, not just in the genitals.

1

FOUR
THINGS
=== THAT WILL ===
REVOLUTIONIZE
YOUR SEX LIFE

IF YOU DO NOTHING ELSE but read the first chapter of this book, I'll be happy.

That's because it focuses on the single most important factor that will determine whether or not you are happy sexually, whatever your age: the way you think about sex. Changing how you think is as powerful as changing how you behave, perhaps even more so.

Knowledge, as always, is power. It's far more important to understand the fundamentals of how your body and desire work than it is to master a new technique. Not that variety and effective sex skills aren't important—they are. It's just that they're utterly useless unless your head's in the right place.

I'll be expanding on everything I touch on here as the book progresses, but if you take these four fundamental principles on board now, the rest is easy.

❶ MANAGE YOUR EXPECTATIONS

We all look wistfully back at the sex we had when we were 18, and there isn't a couple alive who wouldn't turn back time (and freeze it) to relive the enthusiastic, lusty sex they had in that first year of being together. But who says that "good sex" has to conform to the cliché of the frantic, energetic coupling of young bodies with desire ignited by merely a glance? For many couples, the kind of sex you have later in life can turn out to be far superior.

Young sex isn't better sex; it's simply a different style of sex

Our bodies change as we age. Our lives change. What we want from life changes. I don't want to do the same things I wanted to in my twenties, and I certainly don't want the sort of sex I had back then either (all that hard, deep thrusting—are you kidding?).

Sex in your fifties and over is gentler, unhurried, less focused on penetration. One reason why older couples report higher satisfaction with sex is that they slow down and spend longer on foreplay. (Foreplay is necessary at any age, but try skipping it post-50—it's disastrous!)

Genitals age along with the rest of our bodies. While women moan about dry, sensitive vaginas, men lament the loss of the hard, strapping erections of their youth. In their twenties, they got an erection just thinking about sex. Post-50, most men need strong, firm stimulation, and it might take a while.

This is normal. It's called aging, folks, and it's going to happen no matter what. But everyone has a choice about how they deal with it. You can find it all terribly depressing and go down a sad, bitter path, grieving for your youth and focusing on everything that's bad about getting older. Become a grumpy old woman or man. Or you can get a grip, accept reality, look for the positives, and maybe have a laugh or two as you sail merrily, sexily, forward.

It's wasted energy, worrying about getting old. Equally pointless is going on about how great the sex you had at the start was, feeling like nothing has measured up since.

Spontaneous sex is overrated

Spontaneity is something else that's talked about a lot. We never have spontaneous sex anymore. We used to at the start. I miss it.

Are you sure it was all spur of the moment? When they first meet, couples put a huge amount of effort into planning sex. You work out what you'll wear to show off your body to maximum potential, choose underwear carefully, make sure the bed linen is fresh, think about music, lighting, what sort of things you'll do to each other once you get going, how they'll react when you pull out that signature sex move that brought all your previous lovers to their knees. In reality, sex is a special occasion at the start and there's no end of anticipatory planning.

Spontaneous sex is overrated—particularly when you're older. Most women over 50 wouldn't even think about having penetrative sex without some good-quality lube at hand, and lots of men over 50 rely on sildenafil (Viagra) or similar to get an erection. Both require planning ahead. Plus, leisurely foreplay is even more important as you age, so comfort is a priority.

Knee pain and bad backs put an end to any ideas of spicing up that country walk with a quickie up against a tree. Sex post-50 isn't like the sex of old, so stop trying to make it so. Adjust your expectations, move the goalposts, and you might just surprise yourself at what's in store.

❷ STOP WORRYING ABOUT ORGASMS

"We therapists aren't so interested in orgasms," says US sex therapist Stephen Snyder, who's practiced for more than 30 years and counseled over 1,500 individuals and couples. "We're among the few humans on the planet who aren't." An orgasm is just a reflex, he says. Best not to get too emotional about a reflex.

But we do. *Boy*, we do. Women worry a lot about orgasms: not having one, taking too long to have one, why the one we just had doesn't feel the same as the one we had last week—and the list continues.

All pointless anxiety, says Snyder. "Why would anyone worry about how long it takes to reach orgasm?" he asks. "So what if it takes a long time?" And he offers up some simple, sane advice: "Use a vibrator if it takes you a while; that will speed it up. I happen to be biased in favor of easy. If you need a vibrator to make getting to orgasm less of an ordeal, I say go for it." This refreshingly grounded therapist is the author of *Love Worth Making: How to Have Ridiculously Great Sex in a Long-Lasting Relationship*. He thinks—and I agree—that we make way too much fuss about orgasms.

In really good sex, says Snyder, orgasm should be like the dessert at the end of a good meal. Memorable, perhaps, but not the reason you went out to dinner. "The couples who have the best sex are the ones who don't set orgasm as a goal. They just enjoy it—when and if it comes."

Here's someone else I'll be referring to: Emily Nagoski, a sex educator who has written another excellent book, *Come as You Are: The Surprising New Science That Will Transform Your Sex Life*. She is equally as straightforward and helpful—and also wants us all to worry less about climaxing. Distress about orgasm is the second most common reason people seek treatment for sexual problems (after desire), she writes. But "orgasm isn't the goal. Pleasure is the goal." If it takes you longer to orgasm now than it did, that's a good thing. Turn it around, Nagoski says, and think, *Great! I get 30 minutes of pleasure,* rather than, *Why is it now taking 30 minutes?*

She says orgasm is a lot like being tickled: sometimes it's fun, other times annoying, and sometimes it's barely noticeable. "But no one ever asks me, 'Why is it that a lot of the time when my partner tickles me it feels fun and pleasurable but then other times it really doesn't?'" she says. We all know intuitively that there's a time and a place for tickling. There's a time and a place for good orgasms as well. They happen when we're happy, relaxed, in the right headspace, and not feeling pressured. These perfect circumstances don't happen that often, yet we continue to beat ourselves up for not having explosive orgasms, regularly, on cue.

While we're doing some myth-busting: less than one-third of women orgasm reliably through vaginal penetration alone, while the remaining two-thirds are sometimes, rarely, or never orgasmic with penetration alone. If you're one of the many women who've always felt like there's something wrong with you for not being able to orgasm during intercourse, that should make you feel a whole lot better. You're the majority, not the exception!

The clitoris is the "Grand Central Station for erotic sensation," says Nagoski. This explains why 80 to 90 percent of women who masturbate do so with little or no vaginal penetration (even when they use vibrators).

Another eye-opener for some women, perhaps: the clitoris you see at the top of the vulva is simply the tip. It spreads into a vast arousal system, hidden under the skin, that reaches out to your entire vulva and vagina. Much of your inner clitoris is wrapped around the vagina—which could explain why some women are able to orgasm through vaginal stimulation. "So-called vaginal orgasms really just come from stimulating the inner clitoris indirectly through intercourse," says Snyder.

Another thing we need to move away from is trying to label those elusive orgasms (vaginal, clitoral, blended, etc.). An orgasm is an orgasm—and they all ultimately come from clitoral stimulation.

❸ START HAVING SEX

I went to see a gynecologist recently because penetrative sex hurt. "That's probably because you aren't having sex enough," she said immediately. And that's without even asking how much sex I actually was having.

She didn't ask about HRT or whether I'd been through menopause. She didn't impress upon me the importance of foreplay or ask if my husband was particularly well endowed. It all basically came down to one thing: whether or not I was having regular sex.

Use it or lose it

"Use it or lose it" applies to pretty much everything once you get past a half-century, but it's crucial when it comes to sex. Regular sex helps prevent chronic cystitis, uterine prolapse, and incontinence, and it helps with vaginal thinning and dryness. It keeps his erections strong and healthy by keeping his penis oxygenated. In short: the more regularly you have sex, the better shape your genitals are in.

This is the first good reason to kick-start your sex life if it's stalled, or to keep on having sex if you're already having it regularly: physically, sex is very good for you. (When I say "sex," by the way, I don't mean intercourse. I mean any type of sexual activity. It might be solo sex. It might be foreplay. It might be intercourse, but sex doesn't have to include his penis penetrating—ever, if you don't want it to.)

Even if your libidos have flatlined and you're both sighing—not in a good way—at the thought of doing it, there are persuasive arguments for forcing yourselves to have some sort of sex on a regular basis. Research by the University of Chicago showed couples aged 57 to 85 who still have sex rate their general health as "very good" or "excellent." As I said earlier, research suggests the death rate halves for those who report the highest number of orgasms. Sex boosts our immune system, reduces stress, and improves memory. And they're just the physical benefits.

Regular sex brings pleasure into our lives and increases the production of oxytocin, the love hormone, promoting trust, intimacy, and bonding. It makes us feel less depressed and more positive generally, enhancing self-esteem and confidence.

Couples who have regular sex feel more connected to their partner and rate their relationship happiness much higher than couples who don't. Having sex also boosts your libido—and reminds you of how good sex feels, if you haven't had it for a while.

Make sex a habit

So, how much sex do you need to have to reap these benefits? Research suggests once a week will do it. Which means at least some of us need to up our game.

Data collected by a few large-scale studies in the US (published in *American Couples* [1983] by Blumstein and Schwartz) turned up these statistics. Regardless of age, couples tend to have sex more frequently in the early stages of their relationships. Among couples in the first two years of their relationships, 67 percent of gay couples, 45 percent of heterosexual couples, and 33 percent of lesbian couples had sex three times a week or more. The numbers dropped off somewhat with time: for couples who had been together 10 years or longer, 11 percent of gay couples, 18 percent of heterosexual couples, and 1 percent of lesbian couples had sex that often. Let me clarify something at this point, though: if your relationship is in tatters or you haven't had sex for a decade, my suggesting you start having sex with your partner again is on a par with telling you to climb Everest with your hands tied behind your back. (More on how to deal with anger and/or sexless marriages later.) This advice is directed at the average couple who prioritizes the whole wine/sofa/TV thing over sex. Yes, relaxing together is what being a couple is all about. But having sex is, too.

Regular sex is a habit. If you make it part of your routine—something you do and don't even think about not doing, like brushing your teeth—your sex life will last way beyond those who have "special occasion sex."

Desire isn't the only motivation for sex

In long-term relationships, it's unrealistic and naïve to think that every time you have sex, both of you will want to do it. What couples often do is agree to sometimes have sex with each other when it's not top of their list of things they want to do, but is for their partner. It's all part of keeping each other happy sexually.

Enthusiasm is a fine substitute for lust, and once you're into it, desire often ignites. There's a high likelihood that by letting yourself be sexually stimulated, it will trigger desire. Plenty of us also get aroused by watching our partner get turned on.

In my experience, couples who have regular sex say about 20 to 25 percent of their sex sessions are done to please their partners, rather than themselves. Some therapists say only half of all sex encounters in long-term relationships are mutually satisfying for both partners.

No, it's not something you expect will happen when you first fall in love, starry-eyed and idealistic about what "true love" means. But ask anyone who has been in a healthy, long-term relationship and they'll tell you it's all part of the real-life tapestry of two people trying to keep each other happy. (I hopefully don't need to clarify that there is a chasm of difference between having sex when you don't always feel like it and being forced or coerced into having unwanted sex. Enthusiastic consent is imperative on both sides.)

❹ TALK ABOUT SEX

A few things shocked me while researching this book—in good ways and not-so-good ways—but by far the most surprising was realizing just how many couples post-50 have stopped having sex and never talked about the fact that this has happened.

I'm not talking about shy couples or couples who don't communicate well. I'm talking couples who talk through every single other thing in their lives, who get on extremely well, would describe themselves as deeply in love, and who aren't prudish. They'll happily discuss changing bowel habits, feeling tired, and other consequences of getting older, but aging vaginas or penises that only fly half-mast are off-limits.

"Do you even know why you aren't having sex anymore?" I asked one woman, aged 59 and married for 17 years. She and her partner hadn't had sex for five years.

"He's just not interested," she told me. "No idea why. I don't think it's an affair. He's just gone off sex. I have too, really. It's not an issue."

"So, you're quite happy to never have sex again with your husband without ever knowing why or discussing it with him?"

She shrugged. "It's embarrassing to talk about it."

Deciding not to have sex anymore is something some couples do and live with perfectly happily. But if you're going to cut out such an important part of your life, shouldn't you at least acknowledge it? Check with your partner to make sure they're happy with what's going on? Talk about how you're going to stay connected and intimate without sex?

Couples who survive and thrive sexually are those who talk openly about sex

Nearly all sex problems can be resolved if you're able to talk things over with your partner. I know, it can be terrifying talking about sex—especially if you're not used to it. But once you get past those first few awkward minutes, most couples find it's much easier than they thought and an incredible relief to finally get all those concerns out in the open.

He's worried you're thinking he's less of a man if he's having problems getting or maintaining an erection; you're paranoid he won't find you sexy anymore if you confess that sex sometimes hurts like hell. It's not just a heterosexual thing, either. LGBTQIA—regardless of your sexual identity or orientation—no one wants to admit they're anything less than perfect sexually.

"My girlfriend is eight years younger than me and I haven't told her half the issues I'm having with sex," one 52-year-old lesbian friend told me. "Her libido is still high because she's premenopausal and comparatively young. I don't want her to see me as some old woman who's past it."

I urged her to talk to her partner; she refused and struggled to maintain the illusion that all was business as usual . . . until she just couldn't.

"We're lesbians but we're also really into penetrative sex. In the end, I had to admit it was painful, not pleasurable, or avoid sex entirely. My girlfriend was amazing about it, actually. Really understanding."

"She didn't run off in horror, then, because your body dared to age?"

"No," she admitted.

The more honest you are about sex with each other and the more you talk about it, the less likely you are to fall into that awful place where you're both avoiding any type of intimacy because you're embarrassed by what's happening to your bodies.

Talking, being able to get reassurance and be honest about what's going on as you age, can turn around relationships and marriages on the brink of breaking up. As I am fond of saying, mouths are good for many things when it comes to sex, but most of all for talking.

BEFORE YOU EVEN OPEN YOUR MOUTH

Know what you want to get out of the discussion. Really think things through before you talk. Is this about them avoiding sex? You avoiding sex? The fact that you're not having sex? Maybe you want to change the sort of sex you're having, or you want to talk about not having sex anymore. Write what you want in one clear sentence. Check that it's easy to understand. Also check that it's worded sensitively and isn't attacking or blaming your partner.

Work from the positives. Talk about what you want more of in bed, not less. "I would like . . . ," not "It drives me insane when you . . ." Say "I love it when you touch my breasts," if they completely ignore them every single time, rather than "Why don't you ever touch my breasts?"

Use body language. Make sure whatever you want or don't want is backed up by your sexual body language. If you don't like what they're doing, move yourself away from the touch. If you do, press your body against them. Moan if it feels great. Lift their hand away from places you don't like being touched and move it to places you do.

How to talk about sex with your partner

GOOD THINGS TO SAY

To introduce the topic of sex: "I love you and want us to be as happy as possible because we're in this together forever. Can we talk about something? I wanted to talk about how to make sex better/the fact we haven't made love in ages because I miss it/ how it feels like you're avoiding sex. Is that something we can talk about now?"

When you want to try something new: "I had a dream last night that we were doing X." (Watch to see what their response is. If they're interested, they'll want details and look intrigued.)

"One of my friends—I won't say who because it's her business—told me yesterday that she and her partner do X." (If they're up for it, they'll say, "Let's give it a try!" If they're not, it'll be, "Who are these perverted people?")

When you aren't sure if they're enjoying what you're doing to them: "Do you like it when I do this/do it here/do it harder/do it softer?"

"Which way do you like it best? Like this or like that?"

"Can I touch you here?"

If you want more of something: "I love it when you do that. Can you do it for longer?"

"Remember when we used to have sex after a boozy Sunday lunch? I used to love that. Let's do it again."

When you want something done differently: "I love it when you do that. Do you know what else I love? When you do X. That really feels nice."

"I love it when you give me oral sex. But you know what? It takes me much longer now to climax. Do you mind doing it for longer? Sometimes I feel rushed."

When you want to use your vibrator while you're in bed with him: I say "him" because put two women in bed and vibrators are less likely to be a problem. It's getting better with men; vibes are now so normalized, younger guys can't help but get with the program—but older men may still feel threatened.

Here's how to introduce one subtly: Tell him you bought a present for the two of you—a bullet vibrator. They're the size of a tampon and the perfect way to introduce a vibrator to a nervous man.

Use it on him first: buzz around his nipples, try it on his penis, his testicles—keep it light and jokey. Once he's a bit more relaxed and can see how good it feels, give it to him and let him play with it on your body. When he uses it on your clitoris, say, "Mmm. That feels good!" but then push it away after a few minutes, before you climax. (Lots of men look like deflated balloons the first time they see how quickly most women orgasm with a vibrator; he slaves for hours to get to the same point.) Keep doing this over a few sessions—letting him use the bullet on you for longer each time—but still don't make it the star attraction by having an orgasm.

You'll sense when he starts to relax completely: that's when you can take it through to the grand finale. It's easy from there to say, "Let's try another vibrator for a change," if you prefer something bigger or more powerful.

NEVER A GOOD IDEA TO SAY

"I hate it when you do that."

"I'm serious, I will divorce you if you don't stop putting the wet towels on the bed. And, by the way, you're bad in bed as well as shit at keeping the place tidy."

"Why don't we have sex as much as John and Jane?"

"How many times do I have to tell you I HATE THAT?"

"My ex used to do it like this. Can you do it that way?"

"Can you hurry up?"

"Let's just get this over with."

"You don't turn me on anymore."

"What is wrong with you?"

HOW TO
AGE-PROOF
YOUR
LIBIDO

BRACE YOURSELF: this chapter is a bit sobering. Here's where I talk about all the things that happen to our bodies as we age. I won't lie—some of it isn't pretty. But what choice do we have except to face it?

The first way to tackle what's going on is to educate yourself. If you know physically what's going on with each other and what's ahead of you, you're in a much better place to deal with it all.

A TYPICAL SEX LIFE POST-50

While there may not be one "typical" sex life after 50, we must all learn to navigate some pretty significant physical changes.

What's happening to your body

You feel differently than your younger self for a reason—hormone levels change and there are reduced levels of estrogen and testosterone. Estrogen is what keeps your vagina moist, healthy, and flexible—the clitoris, urethra, bladder, and other urogenital components also rely on it for healthy functioning. As levels decline, these organs literally shrink. (Told you!)

Without sufficient estrogen, the vagina becomes dry and less acidic. It takes longer to get lubricated, even if you are sexually excited, because there's reduced blood flow, which makes the vaginal tissue thinner and weaker. Elasticity decreases and the vagina expands less—this is why intercourse can be painful or uncomfortable.

Less blood flow also means less-sensitive nerve endings, including those in your clitoris. You may take longer to orgasm and might find it difficult to climax. The intensity of your orgasms may also alter because of these hormonal changes.

By the time you reach menopause, your body is producing about half as much testosterone as it was when you were in your twenties. Postmenopause, there are only small amounts produced. Researchers aren't quite sure of the exact role of testosterone in women's sexuality, but it appears to affect desire and may also contribute to blood flow and arousal of the clitoris and labia, which in turn contribute to orgasm.

Progesterone—another hormone responsible for sexual desire generally—also declines and stops when ovulation does. So that's three hormones that made us feel like sex, slowly but surely trickling down the drain. Is it any wonder it can feel like someone came in and turned the "up for sex" button to OFF once you hit your fifties?

The news isn't much better for men. His testosterone levels also drop, which means difficulty achieving or maintaining an erection, less desire for sex, and reduced blood flow to his penis. This generates the same list of (rather depressing) consequences: decreased sensitivity means it takes him longer to get aroused and he needs a longer recovery time between erections. His orgasms are also less intense, ejaculation is less forceful, and he produces less semen.

On top of the changes that specifically affect our sex lives, you can also chuck in the inevitable generic health issues that lots of people struggle with as they tip into the second half of their lives. There's a general loss of flexibility, possible arthritis, feeling more tired, and lacking stamina. Perhaps a battle with cancer. Men are particularly prone to high cholesterol, poor cardiovascular health, and type 2 diabetes: these also impact circulation and can lead to erectile dysfunction (ED).

Because the frequency and quality of their erections are threatened and they can't climax as easily, it's not unusual for men's sexual self-esteem to suffer and performance anxiety to kick in big time.

How this impacts your sex life

Probably the biggest issue for lots of older women is that sex becomes uncomfortable. "I get lots of 50-something women coming in to see me and complaining that sex now hurts," a doctor told me. "And most don't tell their partners. There are a lot of women out there secretly gritting their teeth during sex."

Between 17 and 45 percent of postmenopausal women say they find sex painful. Vaginal thinning and dryness are the most common cause of "dyspareunia" in women over the age of 50. If sex hurts, women begin to anticipate the pain, which further diminishes lubrication and desire. A study of 1,200 adults by Durex (2019) backs this up. Researchers found nearly three-quarters of women in the UK (73 percent) experience sexual discomfort during intercourse—and 24 percent ask their partner to hurry up because of pain. Only 57 percent of the male participants realized this was happening.

"Women who do confide that sex is now painful can find it frustrating," says UK sex therapist Victoria Lehmann, who has practiced for 30 years. "Lots of men solve their aging genital problems with Viagra. It's not as easy for women and men aren't as patient. When women stop sex when it's painful, it disrupts the flow, which makes men worry they'll lose their erections. This is a big deal to older men."

Here's some more good news: because the vaginal lining is dry and thin, older women are more prone to urinary tract infections (UTIs). That's why I was seeing my doctor, complaining of yet another UTI, which seemed to kick off every time I had penetrative sex. Another reason why intercourse can change from something we enjoyed to our least favorite sexual activity (and more on how to fix that on page 75).

REASONS TO BE CHEERFUL

But—and here's where you can breathe again—while some of the physical changes to our body aren't helpful, there's a lot of positive stuff happening emotionally to counterbalance it. There's often a willingness in older women to finally let go of the self-defeating attitudes we had about sex in our youth.

When I asked women over 50 to describe sex when they were younger, here are the words they used: *ignorant, submissive, boring, sparse, fear-filled, alien, spontaneous, naughty, dangerous, chaotic, urgent, scary.*

And here's how the same women described their sex lives now: *sensual, experimental, loving, rich, varied, adventurous, caring, still fun; I feel loved, wanted, and happy.*

We're less worried about what people think when we're older, which makes us more confident lovers. We're more selfish, less apologetic: we put up with less shit both in and out of the bedroom. If you've stayed in a bad relationship for the sake of the kids and they finally leave the nest, you're inclined to think, "Screw it. I've done my bit. I'm off traveling to find someone new who makes me laugh." In fact, 50-plus is a fast-growing section of the dating market. (You'll find a whole chapter devoted to a new, single you beginning on page 229.)

If you've been happily married for a long time, there's comfort in knowing that change is unlikely. A "looks like we're stuck with each other" contentment grows.

You've generally got more time and money in your fifties—time to focus on each other and explore as sexual beings.

Some people feel fearless the older they get—all those grannies taking up skydiving are proof—and you might find you're both up for trying things that you once saw as inappropriate. Take yourselves off to Amsterdam to check out the red-light district, do a tantric sex workshop, remember how you used to love sex on the sofa before the kids came along, and leave the bedroom for good.

Sex might be less frequent, but the quality is often better. Orgasms feeling different than they used to isn't necessarily a bad thing. As the ever-eloquent Marie de Hennezel says in *A Frenchwoman's Guide to Sex After Sixty*, "They no longer have that dark, impulsive, almost involuntary side that carries your whole being like a violent wave, an experience that's more instinctive than aware."

In fact, there's lots of new research suggesting sex actually gets *better* with age. A study by *Health Plus* magazine of people over 45 found older women were more adventurous: 89 percent of women admitted liking various positions and locations. Most said sex was better in their forties than in their twenties. Another recent study (2019, the University of Manchester) found 80 percent of sexually active men over 50 are satisfied with their sex lives up until their ninth decade. Eighty-five percent of sexually active women aged 50 to 69 said the same.

Please don't panic or despair if you're reading all this positive information and thinking: *I don't feel like that. Sex is awful for me. This is even worse than I thought.* Research is research: you can find negative and positive for anything, if you look for it. Having depressed the hell out of you with all that talk about bone-dry vaginas and limp penises, I just thought I'd better brighten things up a bit!

If you've gone off sex, for whatever reason, you're not alone. Not being interested in sex is twice as common in women as it is in men as we age. This is probably because sex often becomes uncomfortable and painful for us and lots of couples think of sex purely as intercourse. There are obviously a host of other reasons as well.

I'm going to talk about all of this throughout the book and give you workable solutions that might fix any problems you're experiencing that are adversely affecting your sex life. There's also a chapter on sexless marriages (beginning on page 179) and how to make that work as well, if you decide sex is over for you.

MEDICATIONS THAT CAN CAUSE SEX PROBLEMS

Lots of medications contribute to sex problems because they affect the production of hormones or blood flow, which interferes with desire, arousal, and the health of our genitals. If you're taking any of the following and having problems, it's worth having a chat with your doctor about alternatives or lowering the dose. (This list isn't exhaustive, but it covers some of the main medication groups.) It hopefully goes without saying that you should never stop taking a medication without seeking medical advice first. A numb clitoris might be frustrating, but it's not worth risking your life for.

Antidepressants
Antihistamines

Blood-pressure medications

Cholesterol-lowering drugs like statins and fibrates

Pain-management medication, especially opiates

Diuretics

Heart medications

Beta blockers

Tranquilizers

Antifungals

Drugs used to treat acid reflux, heartburn, and ulcers

SOLUTIONS FOR AGE-RELATED SEX PROBLEMS

This whole book is devoted to solving any post-50 sexual issues you might be experiencing, but here are some simple, practical things you can do to start the ball rolling. All will help to age-proof your libido.

Be this couple

My husband and I never talk to other couples on vacation. Or on planes. Like, *never*. But on this trip we did end up speaking with a couple in their late fifties because we were mystified as to where everyone disappeared to at night when the resort seemed in the middle of nowhere. (It turned out there was a whole beach full of restaurants a short walk away!)

I'd seen the couple earlier, holding hands walking into the sea, chatting away while on their lounge chairs—you could tell they got on well. They turned out to be good company: been married for years, ran a business together. It very quickly came out that I was writing this book and they were intrigued.

"We've both got friends who don't have sex anymore and we're like, what! Why?" the woman said. I asked if they still had regular sex and their answer was "Absolutely! Once a week—always have done since we got together."

Now, there's a couple who's got it right with sex and getting older. Regularity is key. They'd both had health problems—and hit pause when they did—but soon found ways around them to resume their weekly treat. The reason this couple isn't plagued by the problems lots of others are is *because* they've always had regular sex. It's the best way to keep your vaginal lining in great shape and the best way to keep his erections strong. There's a healthy simplicity about this approach to sex. They haven't complicated it. It was something they'd enjoyed doing together when they were in their twenties and they saw no reason why they shouldn't continue to do it into later life. Copy this couple. They know what they're doing.

They also did this . . .

Exercise

I appreciate that health issues can interfere with our ability to exercise, but if you can exercise, do it. Exercise won't just keep you healthy and looking great, it also increases blood flow.

You already know how important this is for our genitals and sex drive, but it's also important for our brains. Exercise increases the production of dopamine, which is important for cognitive function. It also strengthens muscles and improves circulation and mood. Staying active out of bed keeps you active in it.

You'll also be trimmer, so less prone to illnesses related to being overweight. Your heart will be healthier (cardiovascular disease can impact his erections), you'll be more flexible and fitter for sex. And you'll feel a whole lot better about your body.

Research conducted by the University of California found that men who did an hour of aerobic exercise four times a week experienced an increase in sexual frequency and sexual satisfaction. The participants reported that positive changes in body image and self-confidence were what made them want sex more and enjoy it more. It's obvious, really: if you hate your body, why would you want someone else going near it? (More on body image in chapter 3.)

Live well

Eat healthily, cut back on drinking, stop smoking, lose weight if you need to (or gain some). By this age, we all know what's doing us favors and what isn't. Take stock and make changes. Ask your doctor if you should start taking vitamin B_{12}, magnesium, and a good general multivitamin, if you're not already. Manage stress. If you're stiff, perhaps do some stretching (if your doctor advises).

Do things that make you happy

Yes, your desire for sex is affected by hormones, but emotions and your general outlook have just as much influence. If you're excited by life or have just met someone you like, your libido is elevated. Try new things, go on vacation to new places, socialize with your friends, look after yourself. The happier you are, the more open you are to intimacy.

Physically prepare for sex

Take a painkiller if you have chronic pain. If you're stiff, do some stretching. Have a bath or a hot shower beforehand. Do whatever it takes to put you in the best possible place, both physically and mentally.

Change the time when you have sex

Experiment with different times of the day. If you're taking medication and it has side effects, when do you feel your best? Plan around it. Switch from having sex at night, when you're tired, to having sex in the morning. Men's testosterone levels are highest then, so it's easier for him to get aroused.

Use sex as a sleeping pill

Sex makes it easier to fall asleep because it boosts oxytocin—the love hormone—and lowers cortisol (a stress hormone). If you have an orgasm, your body releases a hormone called prolactin, which makes you relax and feel sleepy. Sex boosts estrogen levels for women, which enhances deep, REM sleep, and it's a great stress reliever as well.

Get more sleep

A 2015 study (of college women) found the longer women slept, the more interested they were in sex the next day. Just one extra hour of sleep led to a 14 percent increase in the chances of them having some type of sex the following day. This study also linked more sleep with better arousal. Think this doesn't relate to you because they're kids and you're older? Think again. Another study found that, among menopausal women, sleep problems were directly linked to sex problems.

Rethink your position

Tricky backs, stiff joints, knee problems, arthritis, hip issues—any or all of these ailments can make your favorite sex position impossible. It's good that there are many others to choose from and lots you can do to make the originals more doable: like adding pillows to cushion body parts or letting your partner do more of the work if they're better able to. If you're flush, invest in some "sex furniture": wedges, ramps, and other things designed to help make sex more comfortable (see page 177).

Lying on your side is comfortable for most people, so experiment with side-by-side positions such as the Spoon. You lie on your side, he enters from behind, arms wrapped around you. Draw your knees up to allow him to penetrate, then keep your bottom sticking out toward him and your top knee forward.

The X position is also comfy: lie with your heads at opposite ends of the bed and make an X with your legs. He's inside you, each of you has one leg underneath the other's, one above. Clasp hands for control. This one's good for two women as well, with both of you grinding pelvises.

Consider taking HRT

I talk about menopause and painful sex extensively in chapter 4. If you can take HRT (and it's not suitable for everyone), the change can be dramatic. It helps immeasurably to put your body back in working order and to stabilize your mood.

Use lube

Start using it for every sexual activity—intercourse, hand jobs, solo sex sessions with your vibe. If you haven't already discovered it, this will also make a big change in your sex life because vaginal dryness makes sex so uncomfortable.

Use sex toys

They are the solution to lots of problems. They help you to stay sexual if you're single, help sort any erection issues, and provide more stimulation if sensitivity has decreased. (More on this in chapter 8.)

FOREPLAY GETS A PROMOTION

If intercourse is difficult for you or his erection isn't firm enough for penetration, the things you used to do as a "starter"—oral sex and hand jobs—suddenly become the main course. For women, this is the best thing that could happen to your sex life. As I've said (possibly a thousand times in my life so far), intercourse is one of the least successful ways to stimulate the clitoris, which is how most women orgasm.

Because you're both relying more on oral sex and hand masturbation, technique becomes all-important. Which is why I've included this section, designed to help you both brush up on your sex skills, along with some suggestions on how to adapt to any new challenges.

THE OLDER LOVER'S GUIDE TO GIVING GREAT ORAL SEX

I've written this for the person who's going to be doing it, so hand it over and tell them I made you.

GIVING TO A WOMAN

Choose a comfortable position. She's seated, genitals positioned at the edge of a chair, you kneel in front, with cushions under your knees. Also try her sitting on the kitchen counter, with you sitting on a low stool in front of her. Both make it easier on the neck and you can see what you're doing. Or, if the height difference works, get her to stand in front of you and you kneel on cushions in front of her.

She's in great shape and you aren't (or have knee problems)? You lie flat on the bed and she straddles your face, balancing on her knees and holding onto the wall for stability. If you're in the traditional position (her lying back on the bed, legs apart, and you lying in between), put pillows under your elbows and slip a pillow under her bottom to make access easier. Also try her on her side and you between her thighs, her top leg around your neck.

Consciously relax your tongue, neck, and facial muscles. It's easier for you and it feels better for her. Make sure your neck isn't strained and your jaw is relaxed.

Make sure there's lots of moisture in your mouth. Ideally, you'll have plenty of saliva pooled in there.

Start gently, but be guided by her. Some women love a so-light-it's-hardly-there lick, others just find it ticklish.

Don't head straight for the clitoris. Lick her breasts and fondle them, kiss her neck, stroke her thighs.

Once you do get there, try long licks with the flat of your tongue, a fluttery side-to-side motion, or do a zigzag or make circles. Experiment with fast and slow movement, firm and gentle. Make your tongue wide and flat, and gently swish over the whole clitoral area. Pull up the fleshy part of her mons (where her pubic hair is) and make slow circles around her clitoris with a relaxed tongue.

Agree on a feedback signal. It's too distracting to keep stopping to ask if she likes what you're doing. Try a system where you grip her thigh to ask, "All OK?" If it is, she answers yes by gripping your arm. If it isn't OK, it's fine to stop what you're doing to listen to a bit of redirection.

Don't get all weirded out if she wants something new. It doesn't mean she didn't ever enjoy the other way, just that her body has changed and she needs it done differently now. Some women consistently orgasm for years with you doing exactly the same thing, done exactly the same way, then wake up one morning (usually postpregnancy or post-50) to discover it no longer works for them. Don't take it personally.

If your tongue gets tired, move your head from side to side and up and down instead of moving your tongue, or simply hold it still against her and let her wriggle against you.

Grab her bottom, squeeze, and start rotating in big, wide circles. This indirectly stimulates the anal area, adding the extra stimulation she may now need but be too shy to ask for. Lots of women also like a well-lubed finger inserted anally on orgasm (or before), but always ask before going there!

Your mantra is slow, gentle, and consistent. Don't keep switching techniques. Do let your hands roam around to stroke her body as you're working on her.

Settle in. Both sexes take longer to become aroused as they get older. Let her know you're happy to keep going for as long as she wants and that you're getting as much pleasure out of it as she is.

Ask before you insert your fingers. She might not want you to if her vagina is irritated or tender. If she does want you to, use lots of lube, keep it gentle, and start with one finger or two.

Have a vibrator handy to help if you aren't able to last the distance or she's having trouble tipping over into orgasm. Hold it close to the clitoris as you continue to lick, or hold it in place while you kiss her or caress her breasts. She might want you to insert it (use lube if she does), but the majority of women hold the vibrator on the clitoral area to climax.

Sex doesn't have to include an orgasm. Oral sex feels lovely with or without an orgasm. Not all sessions have to include one.

GIVING TO A MAN

Find a comfy position. If your knees are OK, one of the easiest positions is for him to stand leaning against a wall, while you kneel on some pillows in front of him. Or he can sit on the side of the bed while you kneel in front of him.

Kneeling's out of the question? Try sitting on the side of the bed (or another appropriate-height piece of furniture) while he stands in front of you. It's all about height and proportion: use stairs, pillows, or other bits of furniture to align his parts with your mouth. Or try him kneeling over you while you lie on your back, head on a pillow. He supports his weight on the wall behind the bed with his hands. Make sure you're not at an angle where your hand is going to end up twisted or your neck's going to be strained.

Don't stretch your lips over your teeth. It's easier and more comfortable to relax the muscles in your jaw and neck and push your lips out.

Use your hands as well as your mouth. It guards against gagging and it stops those embarrassing bobbing-for-apples moments, which he'll find even more mortifying if he's anxious about not being hard enough. If your gag reflex is strong, aim his penis so it's hitting the roof of your mouth or the side of your cheek.

Hold him at the base of the penis—this keeps the blood inside the chambers and him harder—then put your lips over the head and form a seal. You're aiming for slight suction so there's pressure, without actually sucking. If your grip isn't strong or it hurts to hold him for a long period, get him to hold himself.

Wiggle your tongue over the frenulum (the stringy bit of skin where the head of the penis joins the shaft), as this part is highly sensitive.

Now move into a rhythm of hand follows mouth. Start slowly and gently, working up to fast and firm. Slide your fist up and down, following the movement of your mouth. Your fist closes as you come to the head and opens as you travel down the shaft. Do it well and he won't be able to tell the difference between your mouth and your hand. Most older men prefer you using a hand as well, anyway, because it makes for firmer stimulation. If he doesn't, just grip him at the base and hold.

Make eye contact as you do it. Doing this one single thing sexes everything up nicely.

Each time your tongue reaches the head, swirl it around the frenulum. Twist your hand as it glides up the shaft and over the head. Slow down when you get to the head—it's the most sensitive part.

Don't forget other parts. Fondle his testicles and lick them. Press your fingers firmly along the perineum (the hairless bit between his anus and his testicles) to stimulate his inner penis.

Let him know you're enjoying it. Moan. Make noise. Stop, pull back, and look at him lustily, then start again.

Don't rush. As a rule of thumb, the older he is, the longer he'll take to get to orgasm. If you want to speed things up, pick up the pace and use a firmer grip.

Add other stimulation. He might now need more than just oral stimulation to climax. Try inserting a well-lubed finger anally to stimulate his prostate (see page 149 on how to do it). Squeeze his nipples or try pressing the side of your hand (make an "L"), hard, in between his legs on the perineum. Put your hand on his lower belly and rub slowly but firmly to stimulate the part of his penis that you can't see.

Think about what you're going to do when he orgasms. Don't leave him flapping about at the crucial moment. If you don't enjoy swallowing, simply remove your mouth, keep going with your hand and let him ejaculate somewhere else (like over your breasts).

HAND JOBS FOR GROWN-UPS

As with oral sex, what used to do it for you might not be what gets you there now. Let your partner know and problem solved. (If you're not the best at talking about sex, there are some tips on page 194.)

Be sure to use lots of good-quality lube and don't be scared to stop and add more. If a vibrator works better for you now than fingers, again, don't be scared to let your partner know (less effort for them!). Ditto, if either of you have any problems with your fingers or hands (like arthritis).

GIVING HIM ONE

Choose your position. The standard way to give a hand job is to do it lying beside your partner in bed. This has always been ineffectual—no matter what age you are. Instead, try standing behind him and reaching your hands around. You can both watch in a mirror for extra kicks. Or try him standing and you sitting on the bed in front of him. If you're in good shape and he isn't, straddle him and sit lightly on his tummy, facing his feet.

Get him to show you how he masturbates and copy it as closely as you can. Pay particular attention to exactly where he places his hand and fingers to start and get him to put his hand on top of yours to check you're spot-on. He can then adjust the pressure or pace to suit him.

The basic stroke is to make a loose fist and pump up and down. Or put all your fingers on one side and thumb on the other and pump or make a shaking motion.

If your grip isn't strong, try rolling his penis between two flat palms, like a roll of pastry. Or clasp your hands and interlock your fingers, overlapping your thumbs, but leaving room for his penis to slip in the middle. Lower your hands over his penis, close your thumbs, then slide your clasped hands up and down, twisting gently as you do.

Mix it up. Alternate 10 slow but firm strokes with a quick, firm pump up and down. Add an extra pump each time you do it.

Use a strand of fake pearls, wrap them around your hand or the shaft of his penis, and slide up and down. Use lots of lube and check the "pearls" first, filing any rough edges down with a nail file. This is great if he needs stronger stimulation.

Use a "stroker" to make things more intense for him and to take the strain off you. These textured, masturbatory sleeves slip over the penis. Manipulate up and down, and use with lots of lube.

Add extra stimulation, as suggested in the oral sex guide (an inserted finger, a squeeze of the nipples).

Get him to take over if it's impossible for you to keep going for any length of time. You watch as he does it. Or, if you really want to make his day, lie back and pleasure yourself.

GIVING HER ONE

Pick a position. Lie beside her, if that works for you and your hand doesn't feel twisted. Or get her to sit with her legs spread, then sit behind her, your legs on either side of hers. Then use both hands on her clitoris, or one on her breasts and the other below. Or sit in a chair and have her sit on your lap.

Ask her what she wants. Some women find they want firmer, more direct clitoral stimulation as they get older. Others go the other way and want it even gentler than before. There's only one way to find out . . .

Use tons of lube and keep it beside you to keep adding more if she starts to feel dry. Reactivate lube by adding a bit of saliva.

Start by holding your fingers still against her closed labia and pay attention to how she positions herself and grinds against you. This is how much pressure she wants. Even so . . .

Touch her more slowly and gently than you think she wants. "Too rough" is a common complaint all women make, regardless of age, but it's even more likely to be an issue now.

The basic technique is to position your index and ring fingers so they're resting on the outer labia lips. Then use your middle finger to gently rub the clitoris up and down or in circles, maintaining a slow, steady rhythm. Use the flat of your finger and the whole pad of your fingertip to rub or slide, rather than just the tip. It feels softer and covers a larger area.

Read her body language. If she lifts toward your hand, she wants a firmer touch. If she pulls away, go softer.

Don't put your fingers inside unless she wants you to. Especially if sex hurts during intercourse. Focus on stimulating the outside and clitoral area.

It's the same formula for a hand job as it is for oral sex. Keep the strokes light, consistent, and continuous. If she needs firmer stimulation than she did before, get her to put her hand on top of yours to show you the pressure she wants.

Try "the roll" for strong, direct stimulation. Use the clitoral hood (the fold of flesh protecting the clitoris) like you would a foreskin, moving it up and down rather than touching the clitoris. Roll it between your thumb and index finger to stimulate the clitoris.

3

BUT

I DON'T *FEEL*
SEXY
ANYMORE

FEELING SEXY IS TOTALLY DIFFERENT from looking sexy or wanting sex—they are completely separate things. You could be a Victoria's Secret lingerie model and still not feel beddable. (Google it: I'm not lying. You think you're paranoid about your body? Try having to show every inch of it to the world for a living!) Feeling desirable is an attitude, not a look. And this attitude is extremely important because this alone can dictate how happy you are with your sex life.

Study after study turns up the same result, year in, year out: feeling sexually attractive means you're far more likely to enjoy sex, have more orgasms, initiate sex more, and be more comfortable discussing sex with your partner. A landmark 2012 review of 57 studies spanning two decades of research found significant links between body image and just about every factor associated with sex: arousal, desire, orgasm, frequency of sex, and sexual self-esteem. It's not rocket science: if you're ashamed of your body and think it's ugly, why would you want anyone looking at it or touching it?

No prizes also for guessing what's nearly always behind this revulsion of our own flesh and blood: weight gain.

WHY WOMEN HATE THEIR BODIES

We women are damn good at criticizing ourselves for a lot of things, but none more than our weight.

"What would happen if you met your friends and said, 'I feel so beautiful today'?" This is the question sex educator Emily Nagoski posed to her students. They laughed and said no one would do that. "But how often would someone meet friends at dinner and say, 'I feel so fat today'?" All the time, was the unanimous response.

Women have permission to criticize themselves but are punished if they praise themselves.

We're bombarded by images of impossibly slim, "perfect" women in every magazine and advertisement, show, and film. Youth is worshipped, and aging is the worst possible thing that could happen to you (apart from getting fat). What hope does the average woman have of growing up remotely relaxed about her appearance?

True, there are body-positive campaigns now, but they're up against a brick wall of messages that promote an extremely narrow criteria of what a "sexy" woman looks like. Is it any wonder that we're churning out generation after generation of otherwise bright, successful, educated women with a completely fucked-up body image that's bordering on body dysmorphia?

In my whole life, I've met two women who don't stress about their body. Guess what? They just happen to have been born tall, slim, leggy, and never put on weight no matter what they eat. The rest of us worried about our weight and body shape when we were young—and are still stressing about it 50 (plus) years on.

This is what women told me when I asked how they feel about their bodies post-50:

"I hate my body. I managed to gain a kangaroo pouch after having my youngest, and since menopause, I just seem to be a bit baggy all over. It's not a good look."

"I haven't felt sexy since I had children and my body acquired weight and stretch marks. My husband never gave me any indication he didn't find me desirable—it was all in my mind—but once there it wasn't going away."

"I've recorded my weight every day since I was 25 and I'm now 57. Every day of my life, my mood has been affected by what the scales say, even though I've never altered by more than five pounds in that whole time. My desire for sex is totally dictated by how 'fat' I feel on that day. If the scales say I'm thin, I'll dress up and show off in bed. If not, I don't want sex at all. My husband thinks it's pathetic, and I agree but don't know how to stop it."

"I'm 62 and have friends battling breast cancer. I'm trying to train myself to look at my body and think, *You're healthy and amazing*, not, *You look fat*. Most days I fail."

How you look is making you hate sex

Does anyone reading this know any man who thinks, *I won't have sex today because my beer gut's enormous*? Have you ever caught a glimpse of yourself in a mirror, thought, *God I look so fat and awful*, and felt that passing urge for sex disappear? Hmm.

A US survey, ominously called "Dead Bedrooms," polled 1,000 people between the ages of 18 and 65 and asked what stopped them from wanting sex. A whopping 46 percent said weight gain.

This constant, exhausting, grueling battle with our bodies and faces is something most women struggle with their whole lives.

What a lot of wasted, pointless, toxic energy! How utterly appalling that we treat the extraordinarily clever, efficient, *magnificent* machine that is the human body with self-loathing and disgust. Listen, if you're extremely overweight and it's a health risk, of course you should look at your diet and lifestyle and rectify it. But most of us don't fall into that category.

We're a healthy weight, just not a "model" weight. Our faces aren't ugly, they're just not "model"-like. And if your shape or weight have changed from having babies, what a wonderful reason that is! Pregnancy, labor, and parenting are brutal on our bodies— of course there are going to be battle scars.

What would you prefer? Your kids? Or your old body? (Maybe don't answer that when you're up at 4 a.m. waiting for them to come home safely.) Everyone says the kids.

What would you prefer? A face with no wrinkles because you haven't laughed since you were 20, or a face that's lined from having a great time? Everyone (except perhaps Victoria Beckham) says the latter.

What's the point of beating yourself up about things like this? Writing this made me angry. I hope it does you, too. If you're reading this book, you're probably over 50. Isn't it time we stopped this stupidity? Aren't we grown up enough now? This chapter aims to teach you how. Not only will your sex life benefit from doing it, but your whole life will, too.

Feeling desired is more important than orgasm for women

Research shows women's sexual satisfaction and functioning both increase when they know their partner is attracted to them. One recent study pinpointed feeling desired as the number one thing that turns women on. Researchers surveyed 662 straight women in a relationship to find out factors that made them more likely to lust after their partner. Being viewed as attractive and desirable by their partner was the most significant factor in determining desire.

This means two things. First, your partner needs to know how important it is to tell you—on a regular basis—that they find you sexy and attractive. Not "You look nice, dear" but "You look hot!" Second, when they say it, you need to believe them. Unless you believe you're sexy and attractive, what they say won't make a difference.

Let's look at how to stop being your own worst critic and, instead, be kind to yourself.

WHAT *NOT* TO DO TO FIX A BROKEN BODY IMAGE: GO ON A DIET

Dieting and exercise won't help your body image. The reason is that our perception of our body has little to do with what size we actually are. You can be an extra small in everything and still feel fat and unattractive.

Michael Alvear, author of *Not Tonight Dear, I Feel Fat*, cites a study focusing on models and actresses in the media. They have 10 to 20 percent less body fat than healthy women. They're also more prone to sexual dysfunction than "normal" woman and have lower libidos. Your weight isn't the problem, it's your perception of your weight.

"Women have a very skewed, inaccurate view of what their bodies look like," says Alvear. "Studies show they overestimate the size and shape of their bodies by as much as 25 percent or more." I can vouch for that one. I got the dress for my first wedding made for me by a designer. I wanted it to be completely individual, so you can imagine my fury when I went to his shop for a fitting and saw a dress on a dummy in his window that was exactly the same as mine except two or three sizes smaller. I went storming in demanding to know why he'd created my dress for someone else. The poor guy looked astonished. "But I haven't," he said. "That is your dress. I put it in the window as a surprise so you could admire it when you came in."

"That is not my dress!" I fumed. "I'm twice the size of that!"

It wasn't until he took the dummy out of the window and I put on the dress to see it fitted like a glove that I believed him. In my defense, weddings turn even the calmest person into a frothing mess of paranoia. What I find astonishing now, remembering this and looking back, is that even after seeing "evidence," it still didn't change my thoughts about my body. I'd seen a dummy that was exactly my body proportions and thought it was tiny but still didn't think I was thin!

The fact that we all overestimate our body size by 25 percent means we all have these moments. The start of being kinder to ourselves is learning to believe our own eyes. You might hate your body, but the reality is it's likely to be at least a quarter less hateful than you think it is.

WHO DECIDED "OLD" WAS UNATTRACTIVE?

It's not just our bodies that women stress about—it's any part of us that dares to show the signs of aging.

I live in central London and am surrounded by women in their fifties who consider Botox, fillers, IPL (intense pulsed light), "vampire" facials, and other laser treatments standard skin care. They cost hundreds or thousands but are thought of as "essential": the same as a good cleanser or moisturizer. I hasten to add that I'm not immune. I've had Botox for years and tried fillers (mostly a disaster, occasionally OK). I've also developed a nasty habit while writing of looking down at my hands, which are now veiny and have age spots on them, and thinking, "Yuck, how did that happen?" (Answer: living on the planet for 59 years.) I hate myself for doing it, but I still do.

Writing a book about sex for "old people" (as one young friend calls it) gets quite the reaction from "young folk." A crinkle of the nose, an involuntary "Ewww," or a patronizing "Aw, that's sweet." I can read their minds: Seriously? Do old people still do that? Do they seriously think someone's going to want to shag them?

One of the titles we considered for this book was *F*** Me, I'm 50*. We all loved it because of the double meaning: Christ, how did I get to this age and please tell me someone's going to still want to have sex with me now that I'm this old! It encapsulated how most of us felt—which is pretty terrible when you think about it, given that a lot of us will live until we're 100 and are only halfway through our lives.

Then again, why wouldn't someone want to sleep with us, just because we're over 50? There are many evolutionary reasons why a youthful body is seen as more sexually desirable than an older body: the most obvious is the younger the woman, the more likely she is to be able to reproduce. But who decided that smooth skin was more attractive than wrinkled skin, which tells the story of a life lived fully? My veiny hands tell of experience and years of flying across a keyboard, creating books that (hopefully) help people. Why are age spots ugly and freckles cute?

In the Western world, we make fun of old age. Anyone who's ever tried to buy a birthday card for someone over 40 knows that 90 percent of them will be based on derogatory jokes about body functions failing. Old age is viewed with distaste, and the worst insult you can give anyone over 30 is "It makes you look old." Other cultures are kinder. In Korea and China, elders are highly respected. "Old man" isn't a derogatory term in Greece.

If I added up the amount of money I've spent dyeing my hair (I went gray in my early twenties), I could have a holiday home in the South of France—a very nice one, too! Add to that the cash I've splashed on Botox, facials, and a mountain of face and body products designed to keep me looking youthful, and I could probably have bought the house next door as well.

I don't know what the answer is. But I do know women over 50 can be sexier than, not just as sexy as, younger women. Helen Mirren, Halle Berry, and Lena Olin spring instantly to mind. But so do other women I know personally who haven't had any surgery or "help" and beat the hell out of the Kardashian-style sexiness of today's youth, which is increasingly reliant on Instagram filters and other help.

THREE THINGS THAT *WILL* WORK TO BOOST SEXUAL SELF-ESTEEM

So, if changing your body won't work, what does? You might be surprised. The top three winners are . . .

1. Having sex

Not all the women I surveyed for this book had negative body images. Some of them were very positive:

"My body confidence is actually better than ever. I took up yoga at 50 and now teach it. I practice every day and I am flexible, strong, and slim. I feel desirable and sexy. (Even if my breasts do still sag!)"

"I'm 49 but I still feel beautiful, and why wouldn't I? There's only one of me."

"Having an affair turned my body image around. My husband constantly made snide remarks about how fat I'd become. The reason I started the affair was because this man loved every part of me. I'm the same weight but feel completely different about myself."

"I was a swinger, and it's a great laboratory for body confidence. It demonstrated that I was attractive to lots of men but also because I got to see lots of real people of various ages naked and sexually aroused. A great reality check in a virtual world of beautiful, manipulated, 2-D sexual images. I was a lean but stocky mesomorph with small tits, so I actually feel more womanly and sexy postmenopause at a higher weight with HRT breasts."

All the women who wrote to me who were self-critical about their bodies had another thing in common: they weren't having sex, even if they were in a relationship. All the women (including those just quoted) who were kind about their bodies and believed they were attractive were not only having sex, but they also reported having good, satisfying sex. Having sex improves body image.

Enjoyable sexual experiences make us feel better about our bodies. If our partner clearly enjoys making love to it, it can't be that bad! It's a win-win scenario: the better you feel about your body, the better sex is. Which makes us want sex more, which in turn helps feed a better body image.

Here's a lose-lose scenario. UK research looked at the positions women who had low body confidence chose to have sex in. The most favored (40 percent) was the missionary position. The position that made women least secure about their bodies? Woman on top.

While only 30 percent of women regularly orgasm through intercourse (without extra clitoral stimulation), a lot of women who do get there do it by being on top and in control. Missionary is one of the least female-friendly sex positions, because adding extra stimulation isn't easy and his penis isn't angled toward the front vaginal wall. Low body confidence makes women choose a position that's almost guaranteed not to make them orgasm and ignore the position that's most likely to.

2. Being great in bed

Improving your sexual skills will do far more for your self-image than going on a diet or telling yourself you're beautiful, says Alvear. Women who know they are sexually competent rarely experience body consciousness while they're having sex—even if they do outside of the bedroom. "Sexual competence gives you bedroom confidence. Bedroom confidence reduces appearance anxiety," writes Alvear.

You'll find tons of practical information about sexual technique scattered throughout this book. Don't skip it.

3. Exercise

It might sound like strange advice to tell you to exercise if you want to reconnect to your sexual self, but it's exactly what will help rekindle your desire for sex.

Research by Dr. Cindy Meston at the University of Texas at Austin discovered exercise can significantly increase sexual desire even in women with a low libido. She found women who exercised on an exercise bike had significantly, sometimes dramatically, higher levels of sexual arousal when asked to look at erotic images afterward, than women who didn't exercise beforehand. Meanwhile, past research has suggested that women who exercise have better clitoral blood flow than women who don't.

You already know that good blood flow always means better sex. Exercise is good for everyone. Do it. Hate going to the gym? Head outside for a walk or do a class at home. There are some brilliant free online fitness classes for all levels. Walk, go for a bike ride, go swimming, do Pilates, try heavy weights (really good for older women), take a self-defense class. Your sex life will thank you.

OTHER STUFF THAT MAKES A BIG DIFFERENCE

Be honest with yourself. You have to *want* to feel sexy to feel sexy. Some of you will go through the motions, pretending you're trying everything I'm suggesting in the hope that it will work. When, really, you're trying to prove that nothing I'm suggesting will work to help you. That's just a waste of time.

If you seriously don't want to be sexual anymore, then shift your efforts into making sure your life (and your partner's, if you have one) is happy sex-free. (Chapter 5 talks about this.)

Expect a flicker, not a fire. Some people feel desire as a huge, raging fire in their lower belly, but for most of us, it's more like a flicker than a flame.

If you're waiting for the fire and think anything else isn't true arousal, you might be waiting an awfully long time if you're in a long-term relationship. Most of us experience high-intensity arousal at the very start of relationships, when we're young—and when we're doing something we shouldn't be, like having an affair. It's rare to feel continual, powerful, potent passion for someone you've been with for a long time and are faithful to. It's just not how humans are programmed.

The flicker *is* the flame. Accept it and work with it.

Initiate sex to feel more sexually powerful. The person who initiates sex more often is seen as the "sexy person." Being the "sexy person" makes you feel sexy. Shifting power—changing from being the person who waits to be asked for sex to the person who is demanding sex from someone else—is an effective way to shake a sleeping libido awake.

Take responsibility for arousing yourself. World-famous therapist Esther Perel knows her stuff and is very clear about this: it's not our partner's job to arouse us, it's our own. This might mean fantasizing to get in the mood or during sex. It might mean putting on some music that takes you back to when you were young and up for it all the time. It might mean "warming up" with your vibrator before you slip under the sheets (even better, still holding it). It might mean reading or watching erotica. While we're on that point . . .

Be careful with your sex triggers. A quick word on porn here. I love watching porn when I masturbate, but I also watch it with my husband—for good reason.

While there's nothing wrong with only watching it solo, be careful about setting up triggers that might backfire. I made a pact with an old boyfriend of mine, years ago, to give up smoking.

He gave up, I didn't. Being a heavy smoker (I hate it now, but back then I would have eaten cigarettes if I could!), this meant I looked forward to when he wasn't there rather than when he was. His presence, previously adored, was now associated with not having fun. The minute he left, the fun—smoking—could start.

We split up.

In the same way, be careful about having all the "fun sex"— naughtily watching "taboo" porn while masturbating—when your partner's not around. Otherwise, them leaving to go to work/going to bed early without you becomes a positive sex trigger: you can sneak off for a solo sex fix. Sex with them becomes associated with being dull and boring. Solo sex is interesting and exciting. If you like porn, explore it together. That way it feeds your erotic connection rather than separates it.

TAKE CONTROL OF WHAT INFLUENCES YOU

"No one is born hating their body or being ashamed of their sexual self. You had to learn that," says Nagoski. But you can turn it around.

Here are a few ideas:

Either take yourself off social media if it upsets you or choose just one. The kindest one, where you find people are less judgmental. If you're not feeling great about yourself, avoid flicking through until you do.

Stop reading magazines or looking at websites that feature "perfect" women. There are—thankfully—lots that have pictures of more representative women, in all shapes and sizes. It's actually uncool and old-fashioned to only have stick-thin models in your magazines or online. Boycott the ones that haven't caught up yet. And if you watch porn but feel intimidated, try amateur porn. The body types are more like the average population.

If you have a friend who ridicules your body, ditch them. Be strict. You should come back from seeing friends feeling great about yourself, not shitty.

If your partner criticizes your body, take a few deep breaths and consider whether you're being oversensitive. If you're self-conscious, you might be overreacting: we're usually more sensitive to our partner's remarks than anyone else's because they're the ones who see us naked. If you're pretty sure anyone would take offense, cut the conversation off at the knees by simply saying, "Thanks for your opinion." Then take yourself off somewhere where you can be alone and write down exactly how the comment made you feel.

Think about the other things your partner says that you don't like hearing. Then, when you're calm, tell them you need to have a serious talk. Say, "When you said X, this is how I felt." Then keep going. If you feel you've gotten through to them, drop it.

If there's a repeat after that and you'd like to give them a second chance, issue a warning. One more and you'll walk.

Then do it. If you can't for the kids' sake or for financial reasons, get a trusted family member or friend on your side to intervene and help them see sense.

Chuck out stuff that makes you feel bad. Too-small underwear? Jeans and dresses that make you feel guilty because you never did drop that dress size to wear them? Far from sparking joy. Toss them out and buy clothes that are the right size and that feel comfortable to wear.

Have self-compassion. What would you say to a best friend who was constantly putting herself down? You'd tell her to stop and give her compliments. Do it to yourself. Be your own best friend, not your worst critic.

Write down every compliment anyone gives you about how you look—everything from "Your eyebrows look great" to "You look fantastic in that dress." Keep adding to the list and look at it when you're feeling anxious.

HOW TO TURN OFF THE NEGATIVE VOICES IN YOUR HEAD

You're not crazy: we all hear voices in our heads. They're called *introjects*, and they happen when we internalize the ideas or voices of people who were or are important to us (parents, teachers, ex-partners, partners). Positive introjects—the voices saying good things—tend to speak quietly. Negative introjects—the bad things people have said about us that resonated—are loud, rude, and insist on being heard.

The trick to managing our introjects is quite simple. Just knowing what those voices are—that they have a name and you're not alone in having them in your head—can be incredibly calming.

The other thing to do is to try identifying them when they speak to you. When you hear, "Your thighs are huge," think, *Ah, that'll be Joan, my mother's sister. Stupid old cow. My body isn't her business, it's mine.* When you hear, "You're crap in bed because your breasts aren't big enough" and recognize your ex, Richard, now an alcoholic, think: *He obviously had a clear grasp of reality. Not.* Once you've done this and have a good idea of where these thoughts originate from, remove the power from them by simply refusing to pay attention to them when they talk to you.

Imagine you're sitting on a riverbank and your thoughts are floating past. There's a nice one—the one where another ex said you were the best lover they'd ever had. Give them a big wave, then passively watch them pass by. Go back to reading your book or lying back, looking at the sky. When you see Joan looming ominously, looking pointedly at your thighs, think, *Joan again*, roll your eyes, and resume reading your book. She'll be off and gone down the river in a minute or two. It takes time and practice to master this, but by God it works.

QUICK WAYS TO STOP THINKING BAD THINGS ABOUT YOUR BODY DURING SEX

- **Focus on how you're feeling.** Sex is about what's happening on the inside, not the outside. Focus inward, not outward.

- **Look at your partner, not your body.** Look into their eyes; it's sexy. Look at their body, not yours.

- **Talk.** You don't have to talk dirty (unless you want to). Just say, "I like that," "That feels great," "God, you look hot."

Moan, groan, compliment. Talking helps you have mindful sex: you're in the moment when you're talking, not drifting off into worrying about how you look.

- **Get active.** Move around. Take control. Do something to them, don't just lie back and let them do things to you. The more present you are in sex, the less time your brain has to get paranoid.

- **Fantasize.** If looking at your partner doesn't work, close your eyes and escape into a fantasy that casts you in a positive role. Lose yourself in it.

HOW TO CREATE (NEAR) PERFECT CONDITIONS FOR SEX

Nagoski talks a lot about our "dual control system of desire" in *Come as You Are: Surprising New Science That Will Transform Your Sex Life*. Put simply, the dual control system of desire means we all have *brakes* and *accelerators* when it comes to sex (if this speaks to you and you want more detail, then hers is the book to buy). Accelerators are things that turn us on to the idea of having sex; brakes are things that turn us off. Your accelerators might include feeling more like sex when you're about to ovulate, seeing your partner naked, being in a place you'd like to have sex, or having a fantasy. Brakes are things like fear of preganacy, fear of catching an STI, stress, a bad body image, fears over orgasm or of not being sexually competent.

It seems logical that to make yourself want sex more, you should put your foot harder on the accelerator—come up with more reasons to want sex—but it's actually more important to be able to relax the brakes. You'll get further challenging why you don't want to have sex than you will inventing reasons to do it, says Nagoski. Here's her advice for increasing your desire for sex:

Figure out what your brakes are. Make a list of everything that puts you off having sex. What needs to be happening to feel desire?

Make a plan about how to turn off your brakes. If you know stress is a big factor for making you avoid sex, figure out how to decrease it. If you're worried your kids will hear, use babysitters, friends, and family to give you both time alone, or go away for the occasional weekend. Be as detailed and specific with your ideas as possible.

A lot of our "offs" have nothing to do with sex. Be kind and gentle with them and give them what they need, says Nagoski. Tired? Get more sleep. Stressed? Find release by crying, shouting, running, fixing the problem. Feeling insecure in your relationship? Let your partner know and get help if you need it by going to see a good therapist.

Assume you'll hit problems. The more you anticipate barriers, the less chance there is that the whole plan will collapse. Don't wing it, Nagoski says, when trying to turn off your "offs." Anticipate problems and come up with contingency plans.

Also try this . . .

Make over your bedroom. Use soft and low-wattage lighting. Try putting glass-encased scented candles on the floor. Candles are proven to change your mood. Great-quality bed linen helps you sleep; fresh air makes you feel more energetic. Hang an erotic print on the wall, make sure your bed is firm enough for sex, and have lots of firm pillows on hand, too, to slip under bottoms and other body parts. Tablets and phones turned off, no TV, no clutter, no piles of dirty laundry.

Have sex *before* you go out to dinner, not after. Who wants to expose their bods when they've got a belly full of food?

Cover up if you want to. Half-dressed is sometimes sexier than naked. If you're really uncomfortable about a particular body part—like your tummy—conceal it. But not by keeping on your T-shirt. Flared, baby-doll style nighties and camisoles do a great job of making you feel less self-conscious but still look glam. Better still, grab his shirt once he's taken it off and wear it during sex, half open, or dare to bare all and choose a position where you can lean on big pillows.

Add some "sex heels." It's impossible not to feel seductive when you're naked or in great lingerie teamed with high heels. Those sky-high numbers you know you'll never wear weren't a waste of money after all!

THE MOTHER-F*CKER

THAT IS

MENOPAUSE

* Well, it's a motherf*cker for some.

THERE I AM, DOING SOME grocery shopping, and a little old lady is in front of me, dithering around and moving at a snail's pace. I have about five minutes to do an hour's worth of shopping. I smile patiently as she peers at a package of flour for what seems like *hours*, blocking my way with her cart. Finally, she moves. Then stops again.

The rage is instant and nuclear. I look at her tiny, vulnerable ankles protruding out of those big, clumpy shoes that old ladies wear to keep themselves grounded, and I picture ramming my cart up the back of them. I'm one breath away from following through.

Welcome to my menopause experience.

I am a nice woman, not generally given to running shopping carts up the back of little old ladies' ankles. But, during menopause, I was an angry, hot, frothy mess of irritability. My friends were scared of me. *I* was scared of me. My best friend, also perimenopausal, then menopausal, went through the whole thing without raising an eyebrow, her voice, or a sweat. The only thing she noticed was that her periods faltered, then stopped. I hated her. A part of me still does (OK, a teensy part, but still).

Menopause *is* a motherf*cker for lots of women. For others, she's like a slightly annoying child, pulling at your skirts when you could do without being disturbed. Everyone experiences it differently, albeit with commonalities.

Here are some of the menopause stories women told me:

- "I was in a restroom in a train station and suddenly, out of the blue, had a massive panic attack. I ran out of the stall and pushed through everyone to get outside. I was so afraid and claustrophobic and didn't have a clue what was going on. It turned out to be a symptom of menopause."

- "I hardly noticed menopause. Emotionally perhaps, I was a little moody and sweating a bit at night. But I think mindful nutrition and not overdoing alcohol helped. And drinking lots of water."

- "Ah yes, the big M. It came and went with no real issues apart from hot flashes and night sweats for a few months. And that was it. Except, of course, since then I'm drier than the Sahara, which has caused UTIs."

- "I thought I'd escaped. I'm 60 and have had no symptoms of menopause at all. Was feeling quite smug about it all! Then I started getting urinary tract infections and the gynecologist took one look and said, 'Wow! There's a lot going on here.' I had severe vaginal atrophy. Because I wasn't experiencing anything on the outside, I didn't think about the inside. She put me on HRT and pessaries immediately."

- "My anxiety level—which has always been high—ramped up to unbearable. I'm on antianxiety drugs now because I can't take HRT. When I go off them, it's a disaster. How much of it is menopause and how much of it isn't, I don't really know."

That's just a taste of the kind of experiences women have. Quite a range, ranging from a few months of inconvenience to years of misery. Regardless of where you fall on it, it's likely your life and sex life will be impacted in some way. This chapter will tell you everything you need to know to get through it. And get through it you will.

Look on the bright side: no more periods to contend with. Freedom! Women who have a healthy libido and are interested in keeping their sex life going continue to have strong, healthy orgasms and a happy sex life well into their seventies and eighties (and longer). Think of menopause as an interruption, not your new life, and you'll be fine.

I talk lots about how our attitude and culture affect our experience of menopause, but first, let's look at the emotional and physical symptoms you may—or may not—be in for.

A LOT DEPENDS ON HOW HEALTHY YOU ARE AND YOUR DIET

It's very common for women to arrive at midlife, when menopause happens, with all sorts of other health problems. We're very good at running ourselves into the ground. We look after our partners and our kids, and try to be everything to everyone and do everything for everyone—often at the expense of our own health.

If you're already suffering from nutritional deficiencies, carrying extra weight, not eating well, and not getting enough exercise, this will exacerbate menopause and perimenopausal symptoms. It's also not uncommon for women over 50 to be struggling with self-esteem issues and depression. A poll of 2,000 women aged 50 and above by Healthspan (2019) found low levels of confidence were leaving a third of those polled feeling depressed, while another 34 percent had experienced increased anxiety.

Hormone levels—held largely responsible for the side effects of menopause—are significantly influenced by how we eat, sleep, and exercise, and many studies have shown a direct relationship between menopausal symptoms and diet, as well as cultural differences. An anthropological study of 480 Indian women found most complained of no symptoms other than changes in their menstrual cycle. Other research found hot flashes are rare for Japanese women. The high amount of soy in the average Japanese diet may well be responsible for this. It's clear that diet and lifestyle certainly play their part.

HOT FLASHES AND VAGINAL DRYNESS: THE PHYSICAL SYMPTOMS

But even if you are in the peak of health, it's the luck of the draw. My gynecologist told me either you sail through the early part, with little PMS and light periods all your life, and then get hit hard by menopause, or you suffer at the start and hardly notice the end. I fell into the first category.

It sounds so innocent. Menopause occurs when a woman stops having periods (for 12 months) and can no longer become pregnant. There's reduced hormone production from the ovaries, which means reduced hormones in our blood. It's a natural part of aging that occurs in most women, usually between the ages of 45 and 55. Except, to many women, it doesn't feel natural.

Common symptoms include:

Hot flashes and night sweats. "It was as if my body's thermostat had gone haywire. I was having overwhelming flashes maybe 10 to 20 times a day. It wasn't something I could pretend wasn't happening, either. It was embarrassing at times, but something I had to get used to."

Vaginal dryness and irritation. Low or no estrogen means a decrease in blood circulation. The vaginal walls get thinner and less elastic, and natural lubrication stops.

The drier you are, the more prone you become to infections, particularly UTIs. This, of course, also means you may experience painful penetrative sex.

Losing the desire for sex or becoming slower to become aroused. During perimenopause, estrogen levels fluctuate and become unpredictable, progesterone production stops because there are no ovulation cycles, and testosterone, which peaks in our twenties, drops by half—all of which can result in lower sex drive. Decreased blood flow means less sensitivity, which can also lead to difficulties reaching orgasm.

Incontinence. Estrogen helps keep our bladder and urethra functioning properly. Without a good supply, pelvic floor muscles weaken.

Problems sleeping. Progesterone helps us fall into a deep sleep. Because our levels of this hormone drop, our sleep pattern is altered. Night sweats wake us up, and higher levels of anxiety stop us falling to sleep.

Yes, that is all rather depressing. But what makes these symptoms *feel* worse is that menopause makes us feel unattractive. In Western cultures, we're taught to link the end of our fertility cycle with emotive, degrading words like "barren," "dried up," "old." Needless to say, this does little for our sexual self-esteem. In fact, there's compelling evidence to say low sexual desire postmenopause actually has little to do with hormones and a lot to do with our attitude toward the changes we experience.

Researchers tested six hormonal factors to determine which predicted more or less sexual dysfunction in women with low desire. Guess what? Not one of them was significantly predictive. Stress, self-worth, trauma history, relationship satisfaction, and other emotional factors have far more influence on a woman's sexual desire than any hormone.

Your hormone levels certainly drop, that's a fact, but the perception that this means the end of a happy sex life is fiction.

BRAIN FOG, NO SLEEP, AND FEELING LIKE YOU'RE LOSING IT: THE EMOTIONAL SYMPTOMS

For a start, the physical symptoms you're experiencing take their toll. Not getting enough sleep makes anyone crazy and hot flashes wear you out. Here are some of the more common emotional symptoms that make menopause so delightful:

Brain fog. Six out of 10 women experience confusion or forgetfulness, mainly in the first year after their periods stop.

Feeling sad, crying easily, depression, feeling frustrated and irritated—or angry to the point of rage—and heightened levels of anxiety and stress. "I thought I was going crazy. I couldn't face anything. I'm a successful freelancer but the thought of going for an interview for a job was beyond me. I basically stayed inside for about three months. My doctor put me on HRT, and only then did I feel myself return to normal."

Mood swings. Lowered levels of estrogen and progesterone influence the production of serotonin, which regulates your mood. This makes your emotions less predictable, more extreme, and more likely to undergo quick, unpredictable changes. "I could go within seconds from crying over a toilet paper commercial with puppies in it to incandescent rage if my girlfriend left the milk out."

"My partner and kids would probably say that my mood was a bit labile, but I would say that they were just pissing me off!"

TREATMENTS THAT WILL
GET YOU THROUGH

The treatment you seek will depend on the symptoms you're experiencing, current and past health conditions, and risk factors, but this is a good basic plan to follow if you feel you need a bit of help.

Consider getting a vaginal and pelvic examination

It's not typically required for you to start any treatment, so if you don't want to, it's fine to verbally report any symptoms. But it will tell you what shape you're in and what you need to be aware of. Get into the habit of getting regular screenings: they're important for menopausal women. Don't skip essential breast and cervical screenings.

Consider getting a hormone test

Again, it's not required but it is helpful and may give a clearer picture of what's going on and dictate the treatment you require.

Consider taking HRT

Studies about the side effects of HRT continue. Some maintain the benefits of symptom relief outweigh the possible dangers, while other reports say the opposite. Whether you take it is an individual choice that absolutely depends on your personal health history as well as other factors. There are women who absolutely shouldn't take HRT—if you have current or suspected breast cancer, have had a blood clot and are not on treatment, for instance—but many can. And wow does it make a difference if you can.

For me, within a week of taking it, I could feel the world righting on its axis. My skin glowed again, my mood leveled, my rages floated off into the ether. All of my friends who take HRT report similar results: all good. HRT keeps the genitals in better condition, increases desire and vaginal lubrication—all of which make sex a hell of a lot more appealing!

You can reduce the health risks by taking the lowest dose you possibly can for the shortest period of time, though plenty of gynecologists will advise you to continue taking a low dose for as long as you like (providing you're low risk) to maintain the benefits. You can take HRT in many forms. It's available in pill form, but if you use a gel or cream (that you rub into the skin), you have more control over the dosage and can get it completely right for your personal needs. Topical estrogen—using a cream, ring, or pill inserted into the vagina—can help restore the tissue's health, flexibility, and lubrication. (Women with no uterus only need estrogen for HRT symptom control. Women who still have one need both estrogen and progesterone, which provides endometrial protection.)

Estrogen suppositories transformed my irritated, dry vagina into something human again. I'd highly recommend them for the emotional boost of feeling "young" again, along with the curbing of symptoms.

HRT can also improve sleep, memory, and libido and generally make you feel better. Premature menopause HRT protects bone health and often has beneficial effects on blood pressure; for older women it may improve muscular strength and promote better bone health.

Studies show extremely high rates of improvement in dyspareunia (painful intercourse) in women who take HRT, with up to 93 percent of women reporting significant improvement (me being one of them). Between 57 and 75 percent said their sexual comfort was restored.

If you don't like the idea of HRT, or can't take it because you are high risk, there are natural alternatives. But just because something is "natural" or "herbal" doesn't make it safe. In fact, these products can have adverse side effects and dangerous interactions with regular prescribed and over-the-counter medications. Check with your doctor before starting any treatment.

Vaginal moisturizers are safe and help, and some swear acupuncture works miracles to help manage symptoms.

Another alternative is to use bioidentical "natural" hormones. These are made from plant sources and are similar to human hormones. The jury's out on these. In London, they're big business. Clinics that offer them are packed and expensive, and bioidentical hormones are touted as safer than HRT. Problem is, the industry isn't regulated and there's no solid research to show they work to reduce menopausal symptoms and/or are completely safe.

Consider taking a testosterone supplement

If your testosterone level is low—which happens to everyone when we age—the urge for sex can decrease substantially. It's an important hormone, so it's not just your sex life that may benefit from boosting it. Low testosterone levels have been associated with memory problems, heart disease, and lowered bone density and muscle strength.

Make an appointment with your doctor to get your testosterone levels tested and take it from there. (As with everything, there are risks and side effects.) You may be prescribed a gel like Testogel that you rub into the inside of your thigh or tops of your arms daily. You can expect results within two weeks to several months, depending on the individual. Estriol testosterone transdermal cream is another popular choice. (Products and licensing change constantly, so ask your doctor for the latest, safest, and most effective treatments.)

One word of warning though: taking it may change your personality. My testosterone levels were low, so I tried taking a supplement. My sex drive used to be ferocious and it dropped considerably postmenopause. (Like, really dropped!) Within two weeks of taking the supplement, it was back . . . and I wasn't sure I liked it. There's something nice about not being ruled by your libido: there's a calmness. Life is more peaceful.

Low testosterone means you're less competitive, as well as less likely to run off with your personal trainer or nanny. Once my levels went back to normal, back came an old nasty side of me that I'd been happy to wave goodbye to. I did a spin class next to a superfit guy in his twenties, and I was so determined to keep up with him that I nearly gave myself a heart attack! I started feeling impatient (again) and irritated by everyone (again) and a little too energized (again).

It works, but it wasn't for me. I'd rather a lower libido and a more tranquil life, but I do know lots of women who love the effect it's had on them.

Take cranberry tablets

One thing I would highly recommend if you find you're suddenly getting lots of UTIs is regular doses of (super) high-concentration cranberry tablets. There's no evidence that drinking cranberry juice or taking mega doses does anything once you've already gotten a UTI. But researchers think they may help to prevent them by making it harder for infection-causing bacteria to stick to the urinary tract walls. Consciously relaxing the muscles in the vagina after urination also helps.

Other stuff

Because penetrative sex also seems to trigger UTIs, changing your focus from intercourse to foreplay and oral sex helps enormously. (There's lots on how to do this throughout the book.)

There are medications that can also help to reduce hot flashes and night sweats; antidepressants can help if you're struggling with feeling sad, and antianxiety medication helps if you're highly anxious. Cognitive behavioral therapy is another option.

Clinics offering vaginal rejuvenation laser treatment claim to help severe vaginal atrophy and urinary incontinence, but at the time of writing, there was poor scientific evidence for this.

IS MENOPAUSE ALL IN THE MIND?

The symptoms of menopause are not universal and vary among cultures. Some think the culture we live in is *the* most important factor in predicting what your experience of menopause will be.

The Western world idolizes youth. Other cultures respect old age. We think of menopause as an ending, almost a "disease." Other cultures think of it as a beginning, transformative. A time of freedom and respect for women. There's a school of thought that suggests this sense of shame and stigma that surrounds menopause in the West is making our symptoms worse. If menopause were something to be celebrated rather than feared, would it bother us less?

The answer is—of course! If you get a hot flash in public and are embarrassed by it, you're obviously going to feel it more intensely. If it doesn't matter, you do what you do when you're alone: ride it out until it passes. No big deal.

The Japanese word for menopause is *konenki*, which roughly translates to "renewal years" and "energy." In China, the old are seen as wise and their opinions highly sought. Chinese and Japanese women are less likely to have night sweats and hot flashes. Rural Mayan women look forward to menopause because they become known as wise women and hold a place of power in the community.

Dr. Mary Jane Minkin, a professor from Yale Medical School, reviewed results from 8,200 men and women (aged 55 to 65) in North America and Europe to find out how menopause impacted their sex lives and relationships. Guess what? The magnitude of suffering for typical symptoms like vaginal dryness, hot flashes, and weight gain varied by nationality. "In societies where age is more revered, and the older woman is the wiser and better woman, menopausal symptoms are significantly less bothersome," Minkin says. "Where older is not better, many women equate menopause with old age, and symptoms can be much more devastating."

"How it affects you also strongly depends on where it sits in your timeline," says UK sex therapist Victoria Lehmann. "A lot of things happen around that time. Parents die. Couples divorce. Careers end. There are sudden deaths. Some women don't notice menopausal symptoms because there's so much else to worry about." Women in third-world cultures don't have the luxury of worrying about menopause symptoms. If getting fresh water means risking your life to get to a well, a hot flash is the least of your worries.

Then there are the French . . .

The French woman's guide to menopause

There's a reason why there are so many books starting with "The French woman's guide to. . . ." French women deal with a lot of things differently than the rest of the world.

For a start, age is no barrier to being "sexy" in France. Take the current French president's wife, Brigitte Macron. At 67, not only is she 25 years older than her 42-year-old husband, but she's still rocking miniskirts and leather trousers. Marie de Hennezel sums up the French attitude to aging in her usual graceful style: "The heart does not age. An inner youthfulness can be sexier than youth itself."

The second thing French women do is they don't talk about menopause or even acknowledge it. They haven't quite managed to change the laws of nature—their periods do actually stop (*mon dieu!*)—but most won't even discuss menopause with their close friends.

Julie Parker, who is married to a Frenchman and has lived in France for 26 years, says she knows all the intimate details of all her friends' lives. "And yet, when I settled down hoping for cozy chats and confidences on menopause, I was confronted by raised eyebrows, Gallic shoulder shrugging, and answers that ranged from 'I don't remember' to 'I barely noticed.'" Not one out of the 10 or so women she approached was willing to discuss menopause with her, yet she knew full details of all their marital indiscretions.

Another English woman, in a similar situation, reported that when a French friend went to see her doctor about dealing with symptoms of menopause, his main piece of advice was to not discuss it with her husband. Personally, I'm not convinced that not talking about anything is a good thing in a relationship. But perhaps French women don't need to because their symptoms aren't as bad as ours.

Why aren't they? Because they aren't scared to get help from their pharmacist or doctor. A French woman's friends might not know about her dry vagina, but her pharmacist most certainly does. French women are far more open to taking HRT and bioidentical hormone therapy. One trick they use to avoid experiencing anything but mild symptoms is to find just the right moment to switch from taking the contraceptive pill to HRT.

The pill acts as a form of HRT: move seamlessly from one to the other and you're unlikely to have severe, or even noticeable, symptoms in lots of cases. Others just continue taking the pill, even if the purpose changes from contraception to HRT. (There are many other options if this appeals: ask your doctor what would suit you best.)

On the topic of contraception, just so you know, you can be fertile up to one year after your last period (if you're over 50) and up to two years after your last period (if you're under 50). The coil can hide the symptoms of menopause by lessening the frequency of periods or even stopping them altogether, as well as releasing hormones like progesterone.

Of course, the other thing French women famously do is watch their weight. The higher your BMI, the worse your menopausal symptoms, particularly hot flashes and joint pain . . . or so the research says.

Does knowing this help us?

Is this helpful to the average Western woman struggling with symptoms, to be told it's all in her mind? That if we had a little more French va-va-voom and confidence in our sexual allure, we'd manage menopause better? That if we lived in a less youth-obsessed culture, we'd have a better time of it? Probably not. I was healthy, the right weight, still felt sexy, and had good sexual self-esteem when I went through menopause at 48 and that didn't stop me from having ghastly hot flashes, dry skin, a dry vagina, and painful sex. There's no way my menopause was imagined.

A more logical theory is that the world divides into women who experience lots of menopausal symptoms and those who experience only a few. Diet and culture play a part, as does lifestyle, genetics, and our general health and attitude, as well as how we measure our worth in society and how society views us. It's a combination of a lot of factors.

The French don't get everything right. Rather than clam up, I think we need to talk more about menopause. I've taken extraordinary delight every time I've written the words "dry vagina" in this chapter. We need to normalize the term. Say to our friends, "God, my vagina's so dry today. I just know I'm on the verge of another damned UTI!" the same way we say, "I feel so congested. I feel like I'm getting a cold." If women stop being embarrassed by what is a natural bodily function, you never know, the rest of society might follow suit.

WHEN MENOPAUSE MEANS SEX IS NOW PAINFUL

I'm one of the many women who associate sex with pain. (It's better now, but sex will never be as comfortable as it used to be.) Nearly every woman feels pain at some point, in some circumstance in her life, during intercourse. We've all let out an *"Ouch!"* delivered with an accusing glare, if our partners thrust a little too deeply, hitting the cervix. That's easily fixed by changing position and shallower thrusting. But constant, persistent pain is something completely different. Pay attention to it. Never ignore pain anywhere in your body.

The (long) list of reasons why penetration can cause pain

Dyspareunia is the name for any pain associated with intercourse. There are many things that cause it, and an accurate diagnosis is key to treating it effectively.

Don't kid yourself that the pain will just go away with time. It won't. Don't tell yourself you're imagining it. You aren't. Even if it's not acute pain you're feeling, it's still pain. Which means something you used to look forward to (sex) becomes something you dread.

This list of possible causes isn't for self-diagnosis—your first step is a doctor's appointment—but it might help you pin down the type of pain you're experiencing so you can explain it clearly to your doctor. Remember: Dr. Google is not a reliable source for solving health problems. Only a qualified doctor can do that.

Aging and menopause cause vaginal atrophy of the lining of the vagina for all the reasons I'm sure you know by heart by now. In case you skipped those parts, drops in hormone levels make the vaginal walls thinner and drier. The canal narrows, shortens, and becomes less elastic. The drier your vagina, the more irritated it feels and the more vulnerable you are to UTIs and other infections.

Vaginal dryness. We've talked about this a lot before. I'm talking about it again here because it's a big problem for many women.

In an American study, vaginal discomfort related to menopausal changes caused 58 percent of women to avoid sex, with 59 percent finding sex painful and 64 percent reporting a loss of libido. Around 30 percent of women and men in the study said vaginal discomfort was the reason they stopped having sex altogether.

Apart from there being a whole lot wrong with the reasons given (why do we think it's our fault/something to be ashamed of/something men should be allowed to get annoyed about?), it's clearly a top cause of sexual angst.

Tense vaginal muscles can also cause pain. Sometimes it's because you're not fully aroused and need more foreplay. Sometimes it's because you're feeling anxious because sex has been painful in the past. Sometimes it's because you feel angry at your partner and don't want to have sex at all. For other women, it's due to trauma in their past—like having been sexually molested or assaulted. *Vaginismus* is an involuntary tightening of the outer third of the vagina that makes penetration difficult or impossible. *High-tone, pelvic-floor dysfunction* is different. This happens when the muscles that support the vagina, bladder, and rectum become tense and can't relax.

Infections, such as yeast infections and sexually transmitted infections (STIs), make our vaginas feel sore and irritated (see page 256 for more on this). *Bacterial vaginosis* is a vaginal infection that produces a thin, smelly discharge caused by an imbalance of the vagina's ecosystem.

Pelvic pain is caused by adhesions, *endometriosis* (scar tissue), fibroids, and cysts.

Pelvic surgery, such as a hysterectomy, can sometimes end up making intercourse painful, as can some cancer treatments.

Vulvodynia produces a burning pain in the vulva and vagina. *Provoked vestibulodynia* also causes a burning pain at the entrance of the vagina when touched.

Interstitial cystitis is a chronic bladder health issue that causes inflammation in the bladder's lining. It makes you want to pee urgently and frequently, and feels like you're peeing razor blades when you do. (Ah yes, personal experience with that one, too.)

How to deal with painful sex

You absolutely must seek medical help. Never attempt to self-medicate when you have vaginal or pelvic pain.

See a doctor. The first step is always to see your doctor. If your doctor is the sort you know will be embarrassed, ask to see a doctor who is comfortable discussing these issues. Believe me, they've seen and heard it all before.

A good lube may not be all you need. Lube helps, but it's not going to make a scrap of difference in a lot of cases. If you don't think your doctor is knowledgeable enough or if they are dismissive, ask for a referral to see a gynecologist or genital urinary specialist. A good gynecologist can change your life.

See a sex therapist. A good sex therapist may also be useful. Medication or another treatment might sort the physical problem, but painful sex impacts your whole relationship. It makes you nervous about having sex and makes your partner worry that you don't find them attractive. Some men think women make it up to get out of sex.

Always add lube before penetration. If you've run out, don't do it. It's an essential, not a luxury. You could try a CBD-infused lube: a chemical found naturally in marijuana and hemp plants. It won't get you high, but lots of women find it pleasantly stimulating.

Try a vaginal moisturizer. They're different from lubes; you use them even when you're not having sex to keep everything moist and comfortable. The jury's out on whether they work effectively. (Personally, I'd opt for estrogen [or Estradiol] pessaries, if you're able to take HRT.) If you do want to try a moisturizer, go for one that doesn't contain parabens or aspartame and insert before bed.

In essence, ask what's available to treat your specific condition. Drug names and treatments change constantly, so there's no point in me naming specific medications, but there usually is a treatment for most conditions. It might be a pill or cream or vaginal pessary.

Sometimes, though, the treatment doesn't work. In that case, the only option might be to avoid intercourse entirely and redefine sex. That sounds extreme, but actually it isn't. Lots of older couples enjoy nonpenetrative sex sessions more than they did sex that revolved around intercourse.

Other ideas include:

- **Try a vaginal dilator.** A dilator is a tube-shaped device that you use to stretch the vagina. Often made of plastic, they come in different sizes. You start by using the smallest in the kit and increase the size as you become more comfortable.

- **Botox** has been found to be effective for vaginismus because it paralyzes the muscles. One doctor claims a 90 percent success rate, but it's not (yet) readily available and is an expensive option.

- **Use a Kegel training kit** to build muscle strength in your pelvic floor. Again, start on the lightest weight and build up to the heaviest. Insert high into the vagina and then do your usual Kegel exercises—repetitively squeezing and releasing your pelvic floor muscles—around the toner ball.

- **Take time to relax into sex.** Put some lubricant on the head of his penis and use it to stroke the vulva, over the clitoris, and around the opening, to get ready for penetration. Don't rush it; take it slowly. Having an orgasm before penetration also helps relax the vagina.

- **Choose positions** that don't allow deep penetration. Any position where you're in control, like you on top, tends to work better because men often lose control in the heat of the moment. Otherwise, choose positions where you're both lying fairly flat with your own legs quite close together. Spooning sex works well, as does doggy style but with both of you lying flat with his legs on either side of yours.

HOW TO GET YOUR BODY READY FOR SEX IF YOU HAVEN'T HAD IT IN A WHILE

Whether you're breaking a sex drought with your partner or are single and just met someone new, having sex after a long time can be a bit of a shock to your sexual system. It's not just you who's nervous—your vagina is, too! As one woman I spoke with recounted: "I recently started a new relationship after two years of very little sex. The first night we did it, we went wild. When we got up, we were both like, 'Holy shit! What the hell happened?' There was so much blood on the sheets and I was so sore. I don't know why I thought I'd be OK after all that time without sex. Easily fixed though with a good lube, pessaries—and practice."

Masturbate. The first thing to do, to get sexually shipshape, is to start masturbating. A lot. Recharge your vibrator or buy one and start clocking up as many orgasms as you can. When you're not having regular orgasms, the blood vessels get out of shape, preventing future orgasms. If you value them, make sure you have one at least once a week for the rest of your life. (Not too much of a hardship, really.)

Practice relaxing your vaginal muscles. After menopause, it gets more difficult for the pelvic floor to relax, unless you practice doing it. Start now. I'm not just talking Kegel exercises (though you should be doing those, too), but consciously relaxing the muscles around your vagina. Take your time. Breathe. When you are doing Kegels, don't just focus on the contracting but the relaxing as well.

Do a daily massage. Start massaging the internal and external vulva daily: this helps enormously to prepare for sex. Use lube and really push your fingers into the skin—you're massaging what's underneath, so use firm, circular movements. Go over the whole area, including the clitoris and the opening of the vagina. Do this for about five minutes before moving into an internal massage.

Add a slim vibrator. Add lube and slide a very slim vibe inside you. Relax around it. Don't thrust the vibe in and out, move it in a circular motion. Your aim is to stimulate the walls of the vagina, not turn yourself on. You can also simply turn it on and leave it in place for five minutes. If you feel up to it, slip a finger in beside the toy. If not, build up to doing this over the next few days. Anyone who isn't having regular penetrative sex can benefit from doing daily genital massage.

Add estrogen. If you're dry, you might want to visit your doctor and ask for an estrogen ring, which will also help to get you sex ready by upping the flexibility and thickness of the vaginal wall.

You're ready for intercourse when you can fit three fingers inside, comfortably. Use lots of silicone-based lube when you do, have plenty of foreplay, and take it slowly.

TWO LIFE-CHANGING, INSTANT FIXES FOR PAINFUL SEX

1. Change the way your partner thrusts. Ditch the deep, hard thrusting you used to enjoy and get him to penetrate slowly, stopping every inch, to let you relax around him. Once he's fully penetrated, keep your pelvises close and grind together in a circular motion. He can put his hands under your buttocks to lift your bottom toward him. Keep the grinding slow and consistent.

If he's not open to moving away from the old-style thrusting, the likelihood is you will eventually stop having penetrative sex. Switch to a gentler style, and chances are you will keep having intercourse. Tell him this, if there are any complaints or stubbornness on his part. (The reason why I'm not addressing any of this to female-female partners is because women understand painful penetration. It's far less likely to be an issue.)

2. Add a "buffer" to stop him from thrusting too deeply.
You can buy squishy rings that sit at the base of his penis to stop him penetrating deeply during intercourse. If he's wearing a buffer, he can thrust away without having to worry about going too deep, and you can relax, knowing it's not going to hurt if he does get carried away.

Ohnut is one brand: nice and stretchy and formulated to prevent painful sex. It works very well. Also do a search for "ministrokers" or "mini–head strokers" or "blow-job strokers" and you'll see other choices. These are like a normal male masturbatory sleeve (or ""stroker"), except half the size.

SEX AFTER SURGERY AND ILLNESS

This is a huge issue and something I can't hope to do justice to in a general book about midlife sex because there's so much to cover. It's complex, too; it's not just about overcoming the physical side effects of an illness or treatment, but going back to thinking of your body as something that gives you pleasure as well as life. Add fear of rejection if your body isn't the same, particularly if you've battled breast cancer.

First, read chapter 3. It will help reassure you on the body-image front. If you've had cancer, I would highly recommend *Woman Cancer Sex* by Anne Katz (she does *Man Cancer Sex* also). The joy of the internet is that you will generally find a book, website, and/or support group for whatever your particular illness or surgery is.

Here's some general advice that will help you to become sexual again after any sort of illness or surgery.

FIND OUT ALL YOU CAN ABOUT THE SEXUAL SIDE EFFECTS OF YOUR TREATMENT

This can be easier said than done because it's a rare specialist or surgeon who will voluntarily bring up the topic of sex. Most assume you've got bigger fish to fry and it will be the last thing on your agenda (and rightly so, at the time). Others don't want to invade your privacy. If they seem uncomfortable talking about sex with you, ask them to recommend a colleague who isn't. Keep asking until you get answers.

You need to know: when it's OK to start having sex, what you can do to get back in shape for sex, and what the sexual side effects of any medication or surgery are likely to be.

Sexual side effects nearly always include pain on penetration, lubrication issues, difficulties having an orgasm, and erection issues for men. For both of you, it's likely you'll be more tired and have less energy than before, which translates to a loss in desire.

This means you have to think about sex and plan around these things. Ask for pain medication if you need it and time it so it kicks in before having sex. Turn planning sex and anticipating what's going to happen into part of the fun.

TALK HONESTLY TO YOUR PARTNER ABOUT HOW YOU'RE FEELING

Hopefully, they were with you in the appointment when you asked about the side effects. If they weren't, fill them in. Talk openly about how you feel about sex now—and let them know when you're ready to reconnect. Lots of partners won't initiate for fear of pushing you too soon. They're also worried your body has already been through so much, you might not want to do anything physical. Talk through any fears and let them reassure you. Give lots of feedback when you do start having sex again.

PRACTICAL SOLUTIONS

- **Don't think:** *That's clearly the end of sex for us because I can't do X.* **Do think:** *What's the best way to solve this? How can we get around this problem?*

- **If fatigue is a problem,** have low-effort sex where your partner takes over and you lie back and enjoy. Time it for the time of the day when you feel most energized.

- **If penetration hurts,** don't do it. Sex isn't just about intercourse. Oral sex is still enjoyable. So is stroking, touching, and using clitoral vibrators externally.

- **If your vagina is dry,** use lube and talk to your doctor about an estrogen ring or testosterone patch to regain vaginal elasticity.

- **If your vagina is too tight,** dilator therapy can help. This involves inserting very slim dildos inside the vagina, increasing the size as you get more comfortable.

- **If it takes longer to be aroused,** spend more time on foreplay. Schedule sex so you can prepare and arouse yourself beforehand.

- **Sex toys do most of the work** for you both: use them. Vibration can also help break up scar tissue and increase blood flow.

- **Rediscover what works now and what doesn't.** What did it for you before might not do it now. Try the Sensate Focus Program (see page 204) for a sensual, explorative way to touch each other's bodies.

- **If you're nervous,** try having an orgasm solo before having one with your partner.

- **Think sensual rather than sexual.** Sleep in the nude. Massage each other. Have a bath together.

A HAPPY ENDING

This is an inspiring story of sex after illness, told to me by a 51-year-old woman who'd had a whole host of different surgeries (including surgical menopause and removal of an ovarian tumor):

"I felt ravaged—emotionally and physically—after it was all over. And I looked like Frankenstein with dozens of staples all over my stomach. I've been with my husband for years and we've always had regular sex, but we didn't have sex for six months. When I was able to have sex again, we both thought, well, we might as well wipe the slate clean and start fresh. We turned it into a positive thing and started dating again, like we'd never had sex before.

"We went away for the weekend with the idea that we'd finally do it but then didn't on the first night because we both felt too much pressure. We did it the next day instead, with little fanfare, when we woke up, like we used to. I was terrified the man who'd always desired me wouldn't now, with my scarred, ravaged body. But it was wonderful. All is fine and it's even better than it was before."

I LOVE MY PARTNER

=== BUT ===

DON'T
WANT TO
HAVE SEX
WITH THEM ANYMORE

IT'S PROBABLY NOT VERY RELAXING being married to me; I'm always shouting at the television, "What the hell is wrong with these people? Who makes these shows? Do they realize the damage they cause? As if that would happen, 10 years in! No wonder everyone is so pissed off with their sex lives, thinking that's what happens!"

My husband eyes me warily during these rants, but he gets it. I find it utterly infuriating when couples who've been together for 10 or 20 years (or more) are portrayed onscreen as suddenly being overcome by lust. There they are, having spontaneous, hot-blooded, animal sex—on a Sunday morning—ripping each other's clothes off in a fit of passion, inspired by . . . what, exactly? Has something happened to reignite this desire? No! Who does this in real life? Who walks in after a long day at work, in a long- (*long-*) term relationship, and feels the urge to shove their partner against the wall and their tongue down their throat, just because?

The shows and films we watch aren't real. The sex they have on them isn't the norm. (It's not even the exception.) And it's dangerous that we secretly believe it is. A more likely greeting, for most long-term couples, is an affectionate ruffle of the hair and a cheek kiss. For many, that's as far as they want it to go. A high proportion of people in long-term relationships love their partners desperately but have no interest in having sex with them. And they have no idea why.

It's baffling ("The one person I tell everything to and do everything with is the one person I can't talk honestly to about how I now feel about sex") and upsetting ("I worry that everyone else is having all this great sex and we're the only ones who aren't"). There are many reasons why love thrives and sex dies over time. Understand why and—crucially—accept that this happens, and it is possible to end up in a different place. A good way to start is to adjust your expectations of what's achievable with long-term monogamous sex.

YOU'RE PROBABLY NOT WITH THE WRONG PERSON

Don't just ignore those stupid onscreen antics. Park those unwelcome thoughts that swim around in your head, whispering, *Maybe this is all because I'm with the wrong person?* You might well be. But if you think that solely because you aren't having passionate sex on a regular basis and you've been together awhile, it's safe to assume it's got nothing to do with the person you're with.

How many good, solid couples have split because they no longer "lust" after their partner? Most enjoy a temporary lift with someone new, then find themselves right back in the same place, usually wishing they'd stuck with their first choice. Relationships move through three stages: lust and infatuation, romantic love, and attachment. Our brains and bodies conform to this model for a reason: in the third stage, you are stable and calm enough to procreate. (The biological point, after all, of sex.)

It's during the attachment stage when it first hits couples that the hot sex they're having might not last. The first time it happens in our lives, most of us hastily split and find someone new, convinced we've chosen badly. Until, there you are again. *No! This felt different, like it wasn't going to happen this time. Not to us!* But it does. Again, and again. We continue to panic, every time it does, and either split, seek sex outside the relationship, or settle for sexual despondency. The grim reality is that we aren't programmed for passionate, long-term sex. Lust and love are uneasy bedfellows, not best friends. Sex and love hormones battle in our brains, rather than happily share space. Losing desire for our partners is actually more "natural" in long-term relationships than continuing to want sex.

Is it a straight couple's problem? No. Gay men, gay women, bisexual . . . this affects all of us, regardless of our sexual orientation.

WHY WE LOSE DESIRE

"My husband feels unwanted because I don't want to have sex with him," said one 62-year-old woman. "But I'm more in love with him than ever. He shouldn't feel rejected. I just can't get turned on like I used to." Ask someone under 25 if not wanting sex means you don't love your partner and they're likely to answer yes. In fact, the opposite is true. Loving too much is what kills sex.

According to the *Journal of Marriage and Family*, 74 percent of spouses who are constantly refused sex stay in their relationship because of love. Most of us don't leave when the sex dies, even if one of you would still very much like to be having it. No- or low-sex couples often describe themselves as soulmates. They see themselves as the same. This, essentially, is the problem.

Overfamiliarity and the "sibling effect"

No one wants to choose between having great sex or a great relationship, but it pretty much boils down to just that. If forced, very, very few people choose sex over love.

What we want from love—security, routine, to feel safe, wanted, protected—is the opposite to what fuels desire: risk, separation, uncertainty, novelty, anxiety, and jealousy. Guess which feels nicest to live with?

In *Mating in Captivity: Unlocking Erotic Intelligence*, Esther Perel says the mistake we make is confusing "mating" with "merging." It feels nicer and safer to have "domestic" sex, she says; it's nonchallenging. To see our partners as sexual, we have to admit they are attractive to other people and "jealousy makes us feel uncomfortable. Our partner wanting us also means we have to make an effort."

Couples who are best friends, who know everything about each other, do everything together—these have the hardest time staying sexually attracted to each other. "Love and desire aren't mutually exclusive," Perel says. "You can have both—they just don't always take place at the same time."

This is central to solving the problem: separate sex from love, and you might just manage to keep both alive. Another way is realizing that women and men are aroused differently. Pay attention: this part's important.

Female arousal is different

Dr. Rosemary Basson was the first to put forward a theory that women and men get aroused in different ways. Men tend to start at no or low desire and move upward toward orgasm. For women, the desire for sex can come after arousal. That's right: after.

Basson had seen clients that, rather than wait to be in the mood for sex, made themselves in the mood by starting to have sex with their partner. Once their body was turned on, their head followed (so long as the woman was willing to allow herself to become aroused). This is called *responsive* desire, and it's very different from *spontaneous* desire, which is how most of us think desire works.

Most people think desire just happens: you see someone sexy, think *I feel like sex*, and hey presto, you're aroused! This "want sex, then seek it" model of spontaneous desire is more likely at the start of relationships, when you're young and your libido's high—or you're male.

Sex educator Emily Nagoski estimates about two-thirds of men have a spontaneous desire style and only about 15 percent of women do. Thirty percent of women experience responsive desire—they want sex only when something erotic is already happening. The rest, about half of all women, experience some combination of the two.

If you find you begin to want sex only after sexy things are already happening, your style is responsive. There's nothing wrong with you if that's the way your body works: it's a normal, healthy way of being aroused. "It just means your body needs some more compelling reason than 'There's an attractive person right there' to want sex," Nagoski says. Yet society thinks of spontaneous desire as "real" and responsive as manufactured—as "wrong" and "forced." Bullshit! It's simply a different way of getting in the mood for sex, and the sooner we all realize this, the happier our sex lives will be. For a lot of women, just knowing this is a major breakthrough.

Arousal is complex, particularly for women and especially as we age. There needs to be a lot of ducks in a row before it happens. "Why do you even need to be sexual once you've got the husband and the kids?" asked one friend of mine, about to turn 50. "Why wouldn't you just go for comfort with your clothes *and* life? Why do you need to look sexy or have sex? Where's the biological motivation? Women need a reason to decide whether to close up shop or try to rekindle their desire. Why should I feel sexy? What purpose does it have?"

Good questions.

DO YOU WANT TO BE SEXUAL?

If you're reading this chapter, you may be at the stage where you could happily never have sex again. Or maybe once or twice a year. My next question to you is this: are you open to wanting to have sex again? Or are you both quite happy not having sex and have no real desire to have sex regularly again?

Not all couples want passionate sex. In my experience, I would say about half of all older couples who enjoy a happy relationship choose a calmer path—they trade raunchy sex for friendship and companionship. They'd rather the closeness of the relationship than the separateness that eroticism requires. (There's lots more on sexless marriages in chapter 9.)

There is no right decision when choosing whether to keep having sex or to stop. It's what works for the two of you. Reading this book, for you, might be about getting permission not to feel under pressure to have sex or a type of sex you're not interested in. But—and you knew it was coming, didn't you?—if there's even a spark of interest, what have you got to lose by keeping your options open while you're reading and making your mind up at the end? If nothing particularly persuades you to change where you're at, fine. If not, what have you lost?

Do you still masturbate and feel aroused when you do? Do you feel a flicker of desire when you fantasize about people other than your partner? If the answer is yes, there's no physical reason for your lack of desire.

Sex therapist Victoria Lehmann has this advice for people considering taking sex permanently off the table: "It's always worth challenging yourselves, one last time. You need to be able to put your hand on your heart and say 'I gave it my all' before giving up on ever being sexually intimate again. You might miss it more than you think."

A DIFFERENT WAY OF LOOKING AT SEX

Let's have a little refresher course on some of the desire fundamentals I've talked about so far. They're highly relevant to the topic of this chapter and I don't want you to miss them if you skipped straight to this part. Don't just read these points. Take time to really understand them and how they might differ from how you think about sex.

Feeling like sex isn't the only motivation to have it. Making your partner happy, feeling connected, reaping the many health benefits, giving pleasure—these are just a few good reasons to have sex. We need to move away from thinking desire is the only motivation.

Desire is more influenced by emotions and outlook than aging. We think of our libido in a medical way—that it's bound to go down with age—but it's actually more likely to be affected by emotions and outlook. Low testosterone does have an impact, as do other hormones, but it's our mindset that has the greatest influence.

Sex doesn't have to be intense. Just OK sex is underrated—people place far too much emphasis on having to have frenzied, wild, all-consuming sex.

"I find it interesting," says Lehmann, "that most women don't mind if sex isn't mind-blowing as they get older. They're OK with it. It's men who can't bear the fact that their wives aren't screaming the place down. But OK sex is fine. Torrid sex had its place in your life span, so does this."

As we age, hormone levels drop. High hormone levels mean high orgasm intensity. Lower hormone levels can make our orgasms feel less powerful. They're softer. Enjoyable, but not sheet-clutching. Again, it is what it is. Relax and enjoy the difference.

WHAT'S THE SOLUTION THEN?

OK, you get it. It's difficult staying sexually attracted to someone for more than a few years, let alone decades. We all need to let go of old ways of thinking. *Now get onto the bit about how to fix it!*

I wish I had a "Hey, guess what? Turns out all you need to fix this is to do this one simple thing" solution. God knows I tried to find one. How to keep lust going is possibly the most important sex issue therapists, researchers, and couples grapple with. I've effectively spent the last 30-odd years trying to find the answer. There's always fresh research, but the conclusion I have come to is this: there is no one solution. Just lots of little things you can do that, together, add up to big change. Things like this:

See your partner through other people's eyes

We all have a subconscious mental image of our partner that we carry around in our heads, based on how we most often see them. Sadly, this is usually dressed in slobby clothes, half asleep in front of the TV, idly flicking through their phone, letting off the odd fart, picking their nails—you get the picture. The rest of the world sees your partner differently: they get the "dressed up for work and play version." The "on best behavior" version.

People are at their most attractive doing what they love. That might be at work, it might be playing sports.

Make a point of seeing your partner at their best. This means getting off the sofa and out of your house. Don't meet at home and then go out. Meet *out*—at the restaurant or park or bar or wherever you're going. I remember three years into my relationship with my now-husband, Miles, watching him arrive at a restaurant. I noticed him as a handsome man before I realized it was him. Then I watched him pick his way through the tables, the odd female glancing up, head turned. My first thought was, *Good job, snagging that guy!* My second was, *Shit. He's too attractive. What if I weren't here and one of these women hit on him?*

Feelings of jealousy and insecurity. Ugh. Who wants those? No one. But they are necessary. When I go through a "can't be bothered" stage with sex, I think about an attractive single woman I met at a party who looked at my partner with (a little too) hungry eyes. "If ever you're done, steer him my way, would you?" she said. I remember her and think, *She could be bothered.*

Staying attracted is about recognizing your partner's "otherness": the person they are when they're apart from you. And yes, this should make you feel slightly uneasy. When people say, "Oh, my partner would never cheat on me," I think, *kiss of death*. First of all, it's stupid to honestly believe this (how can we ever predict where life will take us or our partner?). Second, where's the incentive to keep them interested if this is true? It's giving yourself too much credit (*I'm so fabulous, why would they want to look elsewhere?*) and insulting to your partner. Are you actually saying no one tempting would hit on them because no one else wants them but you?

Look past the obvious

Having just rambled on about looks, it must be noted that the sexiest person in the room often isn't the most physically attractive. So, what if your partner isn't great looking? Attractiveness is made up of many things, and physical attributes are just one dimension.

I was at a wedding recently and watched the most beautiful of the wedding guests flirt outrageously with a very average-looking man she'd been sitting next to. Her husband was sitting next to me and commented, smugly, at the start that he had nothing to worry about there. *That* guy's not going to steal my wife, as if! It was with absolute delight, therefore, that I watched her move from polite engagement to outrageous flirting. Mr. Under Average transformed himself over the course of the dinner. He started out as the short guy, a bit pudgy, gray hair, unnoticeable. But his intelligence, his humor, the way he looked at her and gave her full attention, all made her completely change her mind.

I chatted with her later on (shamelessly eager to find out if I'd read the situation right) and fished by talking about what a pain it was at weddings, being seated next to often boring people. She turned to look at me and said, "My guy wasn't boring; he was amazing. Smart, funny, interesting. If I weren't married, I'd run off with him in a heartbeat."

Spend time apart

Having (hopefully) made you nervous about letting your partner out into the world without you to chaperone, do just that!

Encourage them to go out solo and do the same. Undo the Velcro that's joining you at the hip.

Anxiety over what they're up to is good for sex. Doing things separately gives you things to talk about, which is a tonic for your relationship. Grab back your individuality. Stop being matching bookends. Don't let your partner choose everything for you—from what TV show to watch to what you'll do in bed—and vice versa. Create differences.

Look as good as you can

The better you feel about your appearance, the more likely you are to want to get naked. Everyone owes it to their partner to look after themselves. If your partner keeps themselves fit and healthy and makes an effort with their appearance, how is it fair if you don't and have completely let yourself go?

This means exercising, eating healthily, ditching cigarettes, not being the person who's always the most sloshed at the party. If your partner isn't doing the same, they should be (more on that later). Get enough sleep, do something to relieve stress, smile.

It works both ways, you know, the whole "love but don't desire" thing. How do you know your partner doesn't feel the same way? A lot of people out there do an excellent job of feigning interest in sex that leaves them cold. What you're feeling may also be what they're feeling. Appearance matters—don't kid yourself that it doesn't.

Reinvent "sexy"

On the same note, some women have a strong reaction to "sexy" and hate the idea of having to conform to a clichéd idea of it, particularly post-50. You don't have to. Put your own spin on it.

"I'm more attracted to the idea of natural sexiness rather than painted-on, put-on sexiness," said one 56-year-old friend. "I think sexiness post-50 comes from looking after your body through exercise and yoga and eating well so your skin glows, rather than loading on the makeup and squeezing yourself into skinny jeans."

Stop being boring buggers

We do everything with more gusto when we're excited by life. Do new things to keep each other interested and interesting. Read books that start discussions. Listen to podcasts. Try contemporary music rather than your old favorites. Try a different gym class. Novelty in any area of your life has a trickle-down effect, making us revitalized and more energetic. If you go through life on autopilot, life and sex are humdrum.

At your own risk . . .

Of course, there is another, more extreme way that pretty much guarantees you'll both sexually stand to attention. Have sex that involves other people.

One bored 52-year-old woman wrote to tell me her experience of going to a sex party with her husband: "I read about a sex party that catered to women. I have always been bi-curious but never acted on it, never admitted it to anyone. But one night, my husband and I had the most honest conversation we'd ever had about sex, and it hit me: he was bored silly, too. I laughed and said maybe we should go to a sex club, to make ourselves interested again. It was a flippant remark; we are both jealous people and I couldn't imagine him ever agreeing to such a thing. I wasn't sure if I wanted to do it with him, either. My fantasies about that sort of thing only involved me. I certainly didn't bring my husband along in my head."

Two weeks later, he told her he'd found "something interesting." An "event" being held about an hour away, where everyone had to wear lingerie and sex in public was allowed. "I was shocked but thought, why not? Something needed to happen. I could feel myself being drawn to having an affair and I didn't want to do that. Our pact was that we would look and not touch. But I felt safe there, and we were both so excited by what we were doing that I asked how he'd feel if I let a woman go down on me. He agreed. It happened, he watched, and we went home and had the best sex I've ever had in my life." That was five years ago. The couple hasn't been to a sex club since. "Jealousy kicked in afterward. It wasn't nice for a while, so we decided it wasn't right for us to continue. But the sex we had for a few years afterward was incredible. We saw so many stimulating things that night, talking about it and fantasizing about it kept us going for ages." This may or may not be your thing. I'd imagine most of you will come down hard on the "not" side. It absolutely could damage your relationship, irreparably, going down this path. Personally, I can completely get why doing something like this would work. Would I try it with my husband? No. I would hate watching him be turned on by other people (porn is different), and he says the same. Just throwing it out there for those who might be brave and tempted (more on this in chapter 9).

Try this exercise

CHANGE "DO I HAVE TO?" INTO "WHY NOT?"

This is a useful exercise to challenge your thinking around sex, but before you attempt it, tell your partner what you're doing. This only works if you've agreed to the terms with them beforehand: you'll agree to start having sex in the hope that you'll become aroused, but you can stop if you decide you actually don't want to.

If you don't, you can either enjoy the session for what it was (an erotic moment), help them climax (if they want to and you're happy to oblige with a hand job or oral sex, or let them masturbate in front of you), or let them look after themselves (they take themselves off to the bathroom to masturbate).

Knowing you can stop is the point of this. It means you're more likely to attempt having sex, even if you're not physically motivated. Here's how it works:

Step 1: Answer this: If you had no choice and had to have sex, when and how would you?

On the weekend? In the morning rather than last thing at night? A few drinks in? After a night out? When you've just had a good chat and feel emotionally connected? When you've been listening to music that takes you back to the days when sex was the important thing for you? Identify the right conditions for you and when you might be able to re-create them to try to get yourself in the mood.

Step 2: Come up with three good reasons to have sex, even if you don't feel like it

A lot of you will come up with avoidance motivators, rather than positive things. That doesn't matter. Don't judge yourself on what they are.

"This is about as turned on as I'll ever be. I'd rather do it now than later."

"If I do it now, it's over and done with and I can relax for the rest of the weekend."

"My partner's really up for it and I want to make them happy."

Step 3: Turn yourself on

If your partner weren't home and you were going to masturbate right now, what would you do? Grab your vibrator and fantasize? Read some erotica? Watch porn? Use your fingers and replay some great sex you had in your head?

If you're on your own, go for it—just don't take yourself through to orgasm. If you're not alone, take yourself off to the bathroom and do whatever you can get away with.

Do this and you're starting sex "warm," not cold. Don't worry if part of you is still thinking, *Shit. Do I really have to? Can't I just sleep/watch television/read my book?* Acknowledge the thought and then let it drift away. Keep moving forward.

Step 4: Initiate or agree to have sex

Do this with enthusiasm and a willingness to be aroused. If you want to put a time limit on it, do it: this is sex on your terms. Explore a little. Turn it into a game if that makes you feel less self-conscious. The important thing to do is get out of your head and into your body. Now focus on what you're feeling physically, not on what you're seeing. Just be in the moment.

MY PARTNER'S COMPLETELY LET THEMSELVES GO

What if not wanting your partner has nothing to do with the "sibling effect" and a whole lot to do with too many burgers, beers, and cigarettes? What if you look at your partner and think: *What the hell? They look nothing like the person I married?*

US sex writer Jack Morin says keeping your partner attracted to you is a twofold process. They have to maintain what appealed to you in the first place—his muscular chest, sense of humor, height. But you also need to discover other, new attractive qualities as the relationship develops. He's great with the kids, good at charming your difficult mother, etc. Both are important.

It's not always possible to maintain *all* the initial attractions. If you met at 20, that muscular chest isn't going to look the same at 70. But it's not just the physical aspects that fall by the wayside as we age: the funny partner, who was upbeat about everything, can become bitter and critical if life doesn't turn out the way they expected.

Meanwhile, there are numerous other habits people pick up along the way to turn us off them physically. Heavy smoking, hygiene that's lacking, putting comfort first and wearing awful clothes that do not flatter them—and the list goes on. But by far the biggest turnoff, worldwide and for all genders, is a partner who has put on lots of weight. (I'm talking *really* putting on weight, by the way, not *thinking* you have, which I talk about in chapter 3 on body image.)

Love is kind but it's not blind

So, what do you do if you look at your partner and think: *I just can't go there when they look like that?*

First of all, take an honest look at yourself. Do you keep your side of the bargain and try hard to look your best? If you do, don't feel guilty for feeling angry. If your partner's put on weight through laziness and overeating and is unapologetic about it, you have every right to be pissed off. There is an unspoken vow you take when you decide you want to spend your lives together: I vow to keep myself looking as attractive as I can.

You may well continue to love your partner if they pack on tons of weight, but it's probably not going to make you want to get naked with them. Love responds to intelligence and emotional intelligence; sex is physical. It's strongly influenced by what we see. When your partner really lets themself go, it can feel that they're taking you for granted.

Is it fine to call them on it, then? Say all this out loud to your partner? Umm, no.

If the change is dramatic and he's lost his looks—officially bald, fat, and middle-aged—he knows it. If you accuse him of letting you down because no one could possibly be attracted to him the way he is, this is only going to compound how crappy he already feels about himself. If your partner is female, triple that. Weight gain, particularly, negatively impacts a person's personal body image and self-esteem, enormously. Be helpful, not hurtful.

Is there a reason behind the weight gain? People eat because they're down, and then they get down because they're overweight, getting caught in an unhelpful behavioral loop.

How to approach it

The trick is to focus on health, not appearance. Say you love them and are concerned they've put on weight, or are smoking or drinking too much/not exercising or eating healthily enough. Then offer to help them make changes in their lifestyle that will lead to improvement.

Go for walks and go on a "health kick" together. If they can't kick addictions on their own, make sure they get help. If their clothes sense is what's putting you off, take them shopping or buy something you'd like to see them wear. Load on the compliments when they do wear it. The trick is to reward any positive behavior rather than nag or criticize the negatives.

Tried all that and it got you nowhere? Mira Kirshenbaum, the author of a book called *Too Good to Leave, Too Bad to Stay*, says that people can be perfectly happy in relationships with someone they're no more physically attracted to than they are to anyone else. So long as you still feel chemistry—that there's something about the two of you that's special—it's worth staying.

What is an absolute red flag is not wanting to touch your partner. I'm not talking sexually, I'm talking at all. If you're at the point where you feel revolted by the thought of touching them or them touching you, it is most definitely time to leave.

IF YOU ARE STILL HAVING SEX

Some women don't want to have sex and keep having sex regardless. If you fall into this camp, here's some advice to make the sex you are having better.

Have an honest conversation about what still works and what doesn't. Make sure the sex you are having together works for you. Our bodies change as we age. It takes me longer to reach orgasm, even with a vibrator, and I need this weird combo of soft then hard, then superstrong, then soft vibration. Half the time I don't know what stimulation is going to get me to orgasm, so how the hell is my partner supposed to know what to do if I don't tell him?

The techniques that used to work before sometimes don't later in life. Say, "I know I used to love intercourse but now I prefer oral sex. My body is different." He could say, "I used to not want you to touch me for fear of coming too soon. Now it's the opposite."

Stop being sex robots. This might be more about sexual flatlining—going off sex because it's mind-numbingly routine—than about who you're having sex with. We all have a tried-and-true path to orgasm that our partner knows. Great! If they use it every time, though, that well-trodden path feels about as exciting as your commute to work that you've done hundreds of times.

Develop fantasies and stop worrying about what or who stars in them. You're not attracted to your partner but you sure as hell want your boss? Your partner can't mind-read. Let your imagination run as wild as it wants to, with whomever it wants to. Yes, even that person. It works in your partner's favor in the end. If that fantasy makes you enjoy sex more with them, your brain associates good sex with your partner, making you more open to doing it in the future.

Be sensitive. You aren't the only one feeling a bit defensive about getting old. If you're going to say no, consider your partner's self-esteem as a reason to say yes. If he can't perform as well as he used to, and you reject him, he is more than likely going to think his performance is the reason. (Chapter 7 talks about how overwhelmingly upsetting erectile dysfunction really is to men.)

You love him, right? Again, remember: there are many more motivators for sex than desire.

Don't do trade-offs. Having sex "your way" one time and your partner's way the next seems like a good solution, but it's not. You both feel resentful when it's not your turn and dread the sessions that aren't "yours." Instead, blend a bit of both into the same session. Better still, come up with something new that appeals equally to both of you.

Stop looking at sex as something you do with your partner. Separate it. Put it into its own category: sex. Then think about something you'd like to try sexually. Again, don't think about things you'd like to try with your partner. That's a dead end. Come up with something you'd like to try with someone you're secretly lusting after and fantasizing about. Or make up a fantasy character.

When you do it in real life, close your eyes—don't look at the person you're not into—immerse yourself in the fantasy of doing it with someone you are. Focus on what you're doing, the physical sensations. Don't analyze—experience it through your body, not your head.

Because it's something you haven't tried before, it's likely to hold your interest and get you more fired up than usual. This has a domino effect: your partner gets turned on watching you get turned on. You feel more desired by them, forcing you to see them as a sexual being rather than good old Geoff who takes out the trash.

You may feel horribly guilty "deceiving" your partner like this by fantasizing about another person or scenario. This is a good thing! Feeling uncomfortable—like you're doing something "wrong"—is what makes sex erotic. Embrace it, don't fight it.

This is what we are trying to create. Being unfaithful in your head is completely different—worlds apart—from being unfaithful in real life.

Add outside stimulation. Watch a sexy film or some porn together, try some sex toys. Zero-effort, highly effective.

Don't be complacent. I bet my next royalty check that you put relatively little effort into keeping your sex life fresh. What would happen if you didn't do anything at all to maintain your home? The paint would peel, the grouting would fall out, that door would remain half hanging off the hinge, the carpets would get worn and threadbare. Most of us wouldn't dream of letting this happen. Why do we expect our sex lives to stay vibrant and perky without any improvements or refreshing?

Be selfish about sex. Which is best: the lover who focuses completely on making you happy sexually? Or the lover who gets so aroused by having sex with you that they take their own pleasure in your body? Use you to satisfy their own desire?

This is interesting. Anyone who has read a self-help sex book has absorbed the message that getting your partner to understand what technique works for you is key to having satisfying sex. This is still true—I'm talking a healthy kind of selfish.

Of course, it's important to know and remember what your partner likes and doesn't like. But just knowing that isn't enough. You need spark, emotion, desire to start the engine. "Passion is selfish. Be appropriately selfish. Get lost in it. Don't touch your partner for their benefit, but for your benefit," says Snyder. "Then they don't have to worry about whether you're into it and whether it's taking too long. The classic example is a man going down on a woman. If he does it to give her a good time, she's under pressure, thinking, *How long before he gets bored?* If he does it because it turns him on, then she can relax and enjoy it any way she wants."

Confidence is sexy. We all want a confident lover who isn't scared to take what they want. Tentative, people-pleasing lovers who are too fearful to do something in case it's not what you want or have told them you like make us feel jittery. And annoyed. "For fuck sake, why can't he do something in bed without asking my permission first," one woman married to a lover who prided himself on being considerate raged to me during counseling.

"Have your way with me," I suspect, is a phrase invented by a woman desperate for her partner to rip her clothes off and throw her, face down, on the bed. Couples who get on extremely well have problems doing this. We are so used to taking our partner's feelings into consideration, to not do it seems . . . well, rude. But this is sex, not love. Again, separate the two.

Love thrives on mindful concern. Sex is primal, it's about what your body wants and is telling you to do. If the sex you have together feels like you're having sex with a sibling, it's because you're taking the things that work in your relationship to bed with you. You're neutering desire by doing this. Shift it. Do the unthinkable. Be selfish. Stop thinking about your partner's enjoyment and think about your own. Take, don't give. Screw it if you orgasm and they don't. Worry about them after you're spent. It's a totally different way of approaching sex together. Try it. You'll be astonished at how far this can take you.

THIS COULD BE THE THING THAT CHANGES SEX FOR YOU

This is about role-playing—but not as you probably think of it. It's not "acting out" the plot to a really cheesy porn film. Role-playing is enormously powerful. It forces you to see your partner as someone else. It gives people permission to behave differently. To let the "bad" side of themselves out to play. If your sex life is stymied by your relationship feeling overfamiliar, this could be the thing that helps shift that.

Sex therapist Esther Perel used this technique in her podcast, *Where Should We Begin*. She was counseling a couple who'd both grown up in deeply religious households. They waited until they married before having sex—and then went in completely different directions. The man remained cautious and timid. The woman loved it and was desperate to explore her "dirty" sex side, now having permission to do so. Not surprisingly, he felt intimidated, she felt rejected and frustrated.

Esther's solution was to get Jean Claude—a fictional character who was an experienced French lover—to make love to his wife, instead of her nervous husband. "What would Jean Claude think now? How would Jean Claude touch her now?" Jean Claude was confident, daring, took what he wanted without asking first. The husband loved playing the character, the wife loved having sex with him.

Ask your partner who they'd love to play in bed. Think about who you'd like to be. Think about who you'd like them to be and vice versa. You don't have to stick with the same characters unless you want to.

WOMEN

=== DON'T HAVE ===

LOW LIBIDOS,

 BORED!

THERE ARE THREE MYTHS ABOUT women and sex that the majority of people think are true. The first is that men have a higher sex drive than women. The second is that monogamy is harder for men than it is for women, and the third is that men get bored with routine sex quicker than women do. All of these statements are false. Recent research suggests female desire is completely different than what we once thought. It doesn't like tame, it likes risk. It doesn't want romance, it wants lust. And it's primal. Way, way more primal than society believes. Daniel Bergner, in his eye-opening book *What Do Women Want? Adventures in the Science of Female Desire*, interviews sexologists and scientists who have studied both animal and human subjects and come to essentially the same conclusion. When it comes to craving sexual variety, research suggests women may be even less suited to monogamy than men.

Women do say no to sex more often than men do, but it's not because our libidos are low. It's because we're not given permission to explore our "dirty" side, like men are. Take away the cultural restraints, it turns out, and we'd all be at it like rabbits. With one proviso: the sex has to be erotic and it has to be exciting. Now, how many couples in long-term relationships can tick that box with confidence?

This massive shift in thinking comes courtesy of a new generation of sex researchers who have challenged—and demolished—outdated perceptions. And of another woman, who has no formal training in sex at all, named E. L. James.

THE *FIFTY SHADES* PHENOMENON

If you want evidence that women want edgier sex, think about how many middle-aged women latched onto the Fifty Shades of

Grey series. The interest was savage and obsessive. It might be packaged up in the "rich, powerful man seduces innocent girl" romance format, but sex in the Fifty series is politically incorrect, brutish, and risqué.

E. L. James has sold more than 125 million copies worldwide (and counting), and this is the reason why. Books detailing hot, BDSM sex scenes have been around forever. The reason everyone read this book was because everyone else was reading it. You felt left out if you hadn't indulged—and I'm pleased that women did.

Love it, loathe it, think it's the biggest heap of trash ever written or the best thing you've ever read—*Fifty Shades* got women talking about sex again. Not complaining about partners wanting it more than them—complaining about partners not being sexual enough. It put the woman in the "begging for it" position and, by doing so, dragged sex from the "who can be bothered doing it anymore" basket, where it was lumped at the time, into one that's labeled "Hell, yes!" One 60-year-old woman told me, "I read the first book and literally couldn't put it down. My husband was sleeping beside me, it was 2 a.m., and I was eyeing him up, deciding whether to wake him up to have sex with me. I hadn't initiated sex for years and thought of it as a chore, but here I was, desperate for him to be inside me. That's how powerful the effect was on me."

Christian Grey, the (fucked-up, damaged-but-handsome) hero, became every woman's fantasy, not just because he's hot and rich but because he took what he wanted, without asking. "I'd love it if my partner threw me on the bed and just ravished me" is something I hear all the time.

"He's just too . . . nice. He asks me if it's OK to do stuff. It's so unsexy, it makes me want to scream," one 57-year-old woman, married to a people-pleasing lover, complained.

Therapist Esther Perel famously says: "Most of us get turned on at night by the very things we'll demonstrate against during the day." Women have fought hard to make men respect us—and succeeded, for the most part—and this is (obviously) a good thing. But it's done our sex lives no favors at all.

How the myths finally got put to bed

Research into human sexuality has traditionally been done by men. There have been relatively few female sexologists in history, but once they arrived, they certainly made their mark.

You've probably heard of Virginia Johnson (of Masters and Johnson). Rosemary Basson, who created an alternative model for female desire (which I've talked about), also created waves, as did Shere Hite, who wrote the infamous *Hite Report*. Hite insisted it wasn't dysfunctional to fail to climax during intercourse.

More recently, Esther Perel's *Mating in Captivity* challenged the perception that monogamy is a natural state. Male researchers have also homed in on female sexuality. Jack Morin, who wrote *The Erotic Mind*, argued fiercely that both sexes need lust as much as they need love. Meanwhile, *What Do Women Want?* by Daniel Bergner drew on extensive research and interviews with renowned behavioral scientists, sexologists, psychologists, and everyday women to overturn the myth that men want to roam while women crave closeness and commitment. Wednesday Martin's book *Untrue* suggests that women's biology sets us up to seek pleasure because "women have the only entirely pleasure-seeking organ in the human repertoire": the clitoris.

Monogamy is harder for women than men

The longer a relationship lasts, the more a woman's desire for sex decreases. A German study found that, while 60 percent of women want frequent sex at the start of a relationship, in the four years that follow, that figure drops to less than 50 percent and after 20 years falls to about 20 percent. Men's libido generally remains stable throughout the duration of a relationship.

It's true, Martin says, that women lose interest in sex in long-term relationships. But it's not because their desire for sex is lower than men's; it's because women get bored with one partner more quickly than men do. We're socialized to believe that we've gone off sex, when in fact we're simply craving variety. Lots of men are perfectly happy to have the same sex over and over—it's women who aren't. Women are the ones who crave more erotic turn-ons and who benefit most by exploring porn, fantasy, and the powerful, primal side of sexuality.

If monogamy is humdrum for men, it's even more uninspiring and unstimulating for women. "I used to have two or three partners at the same time. None of them knew about each other and I loved that," one woman in her fifties told me. "The thrill of having multiple partners—the secrecy, the power of having three men lust after me simultaneously, the fact that women weren't supposed to behave like that—was a huge rush for me. Nothing has measured up since. I'm married now and have pledged to be monogamous. But our sex is basic and he's not that adventurous. How am I supposed to be satisfied with the same man from now until I die after having experienced that?"

Boredom is a big issue

US sex therapist Ian Kerner researched 341 respondents in committed relationships: half reported being either bored or on the brink of boredom. Women were twice as likely to report that they were bored in the first year, and in the first three years, of a relationship.

In a study on sexual adventurousness, Kerner found women were significantly more likely than men to have engaged in a wider variety of sexual activities, "indicating that women are perhaps more sexually open than society often constructs them to be." Women were also significantly more likely to have engaged in talking dirty during sex than men, as well as sharing fantasies verbally, reports Kerner.

Instead of being the brake on passion, Martin says, women are the key to a more adventurous and exciting sex life long-term. All we need to do is speak up. And therein lies the problem.

Why don't women tell their partners they want more interesting sex?

Well, for one, they're worried they'll be judged, thought of as "slutty" or not "wife material." I've been writing about sex for more than 35 years, and in that time, I've had hundreds of women ask me how to suggest having more adventurous sex without being judged by their partner. Men are portrayed as the ones who are up for everything and the woman as the one saying no, but it's simply not true.

Another reason why women don't confess to being bored is because we think our partner will have trouble accepting that we're more sexual than they are. "Women shut up and the couple's sex life continues—comfy, predictable, boring," says Francois Renaud, a sexologist and psychotherapist based in Canada. "Sometimes I'll say to a couple, 'I feel like you are masturbating in each other.' Women often say, 'Absolutely.'" It's long been thought that women aren't as "into" sex as men are, but the reality is our sexuality has been repressed. "Slut shaming" is a good example of this, says Renaud.

If you're bored with sex and you're a woman, chances are it's got nothing to do with having a lower libido and everything to do with the type of sex you're having. If we're turning to face the wall, it's not because we're saying no to sexual adventures—we're saying no to formulaic, routine sex. Put something arousing and raunchy on the table and we'd be on it in a flash.

This applies to all age groups, not just women over 50. But when you consider we've been having sex longer than someone in their twenties or thirties, we're even more over dull, repetitive sex than everyone else. This is an important finding for older women because we're more likely to do something about it. We're less worried about what people think and have the courage to tap into this murkier side of our sexuality. Let's give it a try.

MIDLIFE WANDERLUST

Libido loss for older women is by no means a foregone conclusion. "There are plenty of reasons why women can experience a libido surge in midlife," says UK psychotherapist Krystal Woodbridge.

Forty-nine-year-old Karin Jones, interviewed for a piece in the *London Times*, can attest to that. "A sensation took hold of me, vaguely familiar, although distant in my memory: lust. It was as though I'd walked into a mountain mist of desire." Jones was on a country walk at the time. Nothing obvious had triggered it, but she was "suddenly atrociously horny." And it lasted years.

There's a distinct lack of data on how many women experience this unprovoked surge in their sexual desire well after they've had children. (Research tends to focus on what's going wrong, not right.) But it's not unheard of. "A woman's sexual response is hugely stimulated by thoughts, and if she experiences life changes at this age, her thoughts will change, too," says Woodbridge.

Plenty of the women I interviewed could relate to this. One, divorced at 48 after being married since she was 18, had her first orgasm one year later. "My husband was the one who had the affair, but he was absolutely useless at sex," she said. "I was sexually naïve and had never had an orgasm. But I ended up in a relationship with a highly sexual man who gave me my first climax at 49. We did things that made my daughter's hair curl. (I'd insist on telling her—she didn't know whether to be impressed or horrified.) We'd eat food off each other's bodies, we used all sorts of toys in all sorts of places and did a whole heap of stuff I can't even admit to. I loved it . . . When all my friends seemed to be stopping having sex, I was having the best sex of my life."

Empty-nest syndrome might cause angst, but for lots of couples, it brings freedom and time. Time to look after yourself more, to socialize and exercise, and to be more creative. Increased self-confidence has a positive impact on our sexual self-esteem and desire for sex. As Woodbridge reports: "People who have a lust for all aspects of life often have a high sexual desire. If you're motivated, energetic, and have a positive outlook, the chances are your libido will follow, whatever your age."

HOW TO UNLEASH YOUR KINK

It's a depressing reality that we often have the raunchiest sex with someone we don't care that much about. If you couldn't give a damn what your partner thinks of you, you aren't afraid to unleash the less "feminine" side of yourself. If you don't love them, you aren't worried about offending them or hurting them by criticizing something they're doing or not doing sexually. Sex becomes self-ish when feelings aren't involved: both of you worry purely about getting yourselves off, no matter what it takes, and both generally do because of it.

A hell of a lot of couples think married or long-term sex is supposed to be loving and affectionate and feel guilty for craving the "nasty" or "dirty" sex they enjoyed while single (or wished they'd had). But how do you know your partner isn't thinking the same thing?

Being able to get past the fear of judgment and having the courage to ask for what you really want is pivotal to having a happy sex life. Particularly for women. You don't have to like everything each other says or does, or enjoy every sexual experience you try. But you should both feel a sense of sexual freedom and know you can speak up without being slapped down.

Dare to share

This chapter will either be speaking to you or not. You'll either skim over it, thinking, *Hmmm. Interesting. But I'm not really relating to this.* Or you'll devour it in one sitting and think, *Thank God! I'm not some kind of pervert after all . . . and when do I get to try some of this stuff out?*

If you're the former and perfectly happy with where you're at, terrific! But if you'd like to shake things up a bit, dare to do it. You might be surprised how up for it your partner actually is.

A few pointers before you do:

- There are lots of tips on how to talk about sex on page 10. Read those first, if you haven't already.

- Think through exactly what you want to achieve from the conversation. Does it end with, "So that's what I'd love us to do this weekend." Or is it more, "So, as much as I love that you respect me out of bed, I'd like you to be more dominant in it."

- Just because something turns you on doesn't mean it will your partner. Obviously—well, I hope obviously—it's not cool to coerce or trick your partner into doing something they really don't want to.

- Be positive and confident when you suggest what you want to do and be casual rather than make it a big deal. If you're all jumpy and anxious, they'll worry it really must be something out of the norm.

- Make it very clear what it is you want. Is this a one-off or something you want to become a regular part of your sex life? Most people can cope with doing "kinky" things now and then, but few want to do it every single time. The trick is to get into the habit of trying interesting things, without becoming reliant on them to enjoy great sex.

Here are a few suggestions of things you might like to experiment with. One person's kink is another person's normal, so I've started tame and worked up to things like threesomes, swinging, same-sex sessions, and polyamory. Go as far as feels right for you both (but push a little out of your comfort zones—that's the idea of this, after all).

A LITTLE KICK

FANTASIES

Your imagination is the single most potent engine driving sexual desire. Tap into it and you've turned on nature's built-in aphrodisiac.

Fantasies are what keep sex fizzy when your sex life (or your partner) go temporarily pear-shaped. They can make sex with someone we've slept with hundreds of times before seem not only remotely appealing but exciting. Even better, one of the quickest ways to arouse yourself is to fantasize. It's a form of foreplay we can access in an instant: anywhere, anytime, because we carry it with us in our minds always.

People feel enormous guilt over fantasizing about people other than their partner. Park it. Just because you're in love doesn't mean you don't find others attractive: a rich fantasy life keeps everyone happy. You'd be surprised how effective fantasy is for satisfying a sexual itch: think of it as a vibrator for your mind.

Should you worry about the things you fantasize about?
No. The whole point of fantasies is that you have the freedom

to get aroused by something without having to feel guilty afterward. Hardly anyone has romantic, "nice" fantasies.

Should you share them with your partner? I think this hugely depends on what personalities you are and the purpose of sharing. I am perfectly happy with my husband fantasizing about whatever he likes, but I don't have any desire to hear about it or find out who features in his fantasies. Other couples say their hottest sex of all is when one of them tells the other, in explicit detail, their smuttiest, dirtiest fantasy, while they act it out.

Should you act them out? Reality and fantasy are like night and day: totally different beasts. Think about the fallout and the negative consequences first, then consider the benefits, and it's much more likely to end up a positive, happy experience. Don't kid yourself about potential pitfalls. Generally, if other people are involved, consider it risky. If it's just you and your partner, less so, but exceptions obviously apply.

SEX ALFRESCO

Breathe some fresh air into your love life—literally. Having sex outside is a great way to make completely ordinary seem terribly risqué without too much imagination. A hand trailing up your leg while you're lying in bed might be pleasant. But a hand moving up your inner thigh within view of other people is daring. The fear of discovery delivers delicious jolts of adrenaline, turning the tamest sex act into something dangerous and thrilling.

There is a tiny problem: sex in public may be illegal where you live. But it's not like you're both going to strip in your local pub or on the train. Be sensible, assess each situation carefully, keep as many clothes on as possible, and use props to hide behind. A picnic blanket, a sarong, a strategically placed beach umbrella or beach bag, a tent, a tree, a car—all can disguise a multitude of sins.

Dress for sex: wear floaty skirts and no underwear, have a code word that alerts you to someone coming (other than you two), and plan your escape beforehand along with what you'll say. Don't do it if being caught would be utterly humiliating or a nightmare. Full sex is the riskiest. If it's too risky, stick to enjoying some foreplay and finish in private. Some low-risk public sex venues include: your garden, a balcony, a car, a rooftop, a boat, the balcony of a hotel, a swimming pool, a little-used stairwell, public bathrooms with locks in rarely used places.

TEMPERATURE PLAY

Forty-one percent of men and women in the UK are into temperature play, which is based on the principle that you'll feel something more intensely if it's very different from something else.

Anyone who's ever stepped from a hot sauna straight into an icy plunge pool has experienced the effects of temperature play (though not in a sexual sense, obviously). It's been around forever (Christian and Anastasia experimented with both ice-cream and ice-cubes in *Fifty Shades of Grey*), but it's rising in popularity among women.

Why? It's erotic but easy to do—and nipples are a favorite target. The rise in sales of glass sex toys—particularly dildos—is another reason. Glass toys are prettier than other varieties so appeal more to women. Glass also happens to be the perfect material to heat up or cool down and apply to erogenous zones. Temperature play is also about power: one person does it to the other, who is often blindfolded, to increase the surprise factor.

ELECTROSTIMULATION

Would you let an electric current flow through your genitals if it felt good or helped tighten your pelvic floor? Plenty of women are doing just that by experimenting with electro-sex toys. One of the top US sex toy retailers said electro-sex toy sales were up over 100 percent in the first half of 2017.

"Electro sex" is a way of stimulating the genitals and erogenous zones with a safe amount of electrical energy (the human body is mostly water, so it's an excellent conductor). The toy or a conductive pad is placed somewhere on your body (like your genitals) to allow electricity to pass through the nerve cells. This makes you supersensitive to touch and creates sensations that range from a prickle or a tingle to a strong pulsating feeling that causes the muscles to contract.

Why would you want to do it? Because it feels good, it's something new to try with your partner—and because electrostimulators are reportedly great for toning the pelvic floor muscles with minimum effort (and maximum pleasure, if you believe the growing number of fans).

SMOKING WEED

If weed is your thing, chances are you're having better sex than the rest of us. A 2018 study found men and women who used marijuana daily had about 20 percent more sex during the previous four weeks than those who abstained from the drug. (What state their lungs were in is another story.) "Sexual satisfaction was improved, orgasm was improved, desire was improved . . . and pain was better," says Dr. Becky K. Lynn, the lead researcher in the study. Lynn specializes in treating sexual problems in women like low libido, painful sex, and orgasm issues.

Of the 373 women she surveyed in her clinic, 127 used marijuana. (If you think that's high, it is. Missouri, where the study was conducted, legalized the use of medicinal marijuana recently.) Of those who did, 68.5 percent said sex was more pleasurable, 60.6 percent said they had an increase in sex drive, and 52.8 percent said they noted an increase in satisfying orgasms.

Researchers aren't sure why it works, but marijuana is known to lower stress and anxiety. It gives the perception of time slowing down, forcing you to be in the moment and prolonging pleasure, and it also lowers sexual inhibition and heightens the senses, making sex feel more stimulating.

UP A NOTCH

BONDAGE AND POWER GAMES

Lots of us experiment with being tied up when we first start having sex—and most like it. We do it less often as we get older or the longer we're in a relationship simply because it requires a bit more effort than turning off the light and getting into the missionary position. Bondage is well worth going the extra mile: you've just forgotten how much fun it can be! Being tied up appeals because it increases the suspense of sexual pleasure: you can't control when someone touches, teases, licks, or penetrates you and are "forced" to give in (handily sidestepping the guilt that comes with lying back and taking). If you're in the power position, you get the enormous kick of having someone completely at your sexual mercy. Seriously, what's not to like?

Here are some tips if you're into it:

If someone's not sure how they'll feel being tied up, hold their wrists together above their head with your hands during sex or instruct them to keep their hands behind their backs. If they're really nervous, tie them up with toilet paper, which gives the feeling of being held hostage without any threat (at all).

Using everyday objects—like socks, scarves, or old stockings—makes it seem less threatening than serious-looking handcuffs. If you enjoy your first time, then invest in a soft bondage kit. They usually attach with Velcro, which is super easy to put on and take off quickly.

Don't use knots that tighten if the person moves, and make sure it feels comfortable on their end by slipping one finger between the bond and their wrist or ankle before tightening the knots. Keep a pair of scissors handy in case they (or you) have a sudden "Get me out!" panic.

What to do once you've got them tied up? Anything and everything—with a heavy emphasis on tease. Do a strip for them. Masturbate in front of them. Kiss them deeply, then pull back. Give them oral sex, then stop just before they climax. Stroke them all over. Lower yourself on top, then pull away after a few thrusts. Use a sex toy to bring them to the brink, then stop.

Add a blindfold. You can make one out of pretty much anything.

Add some nipple clamps, if they like their nipples being pinched during sex.

SPANKING

If you're a *Fifty Shades of Grey* fan, this will need no introduction. For everyone else, the reason why a well-placed, well-timed slap on the bottom feels good is because of the link between pleasure and pain. Pain is one of the strongest sensations you can feel—and it doesn't diminish once you're accustomed to it.

Some people think it's degrading to spank their partner. Which it definitely is if you don't ask for it and they suddenly start slapping you out of the blue! But *wanting* them to spank you is quite another thing. A lot of the appeal lies in giving your partner power over you or becoming the person with the power. This is where the magic happens sexually: when you swap roles. The person who's the most dominant in the relationship becomes submissive and vice versa.

Where to start? Well . . .

Wait until they're aroused. The more erotically aroused they are, the more likely they are to be up for trying it and receptive to erotic pain.

Start with the buttock cheek closest to you. Run your fingers lightly over their buttocks, tickling them. Then place one hand on one cheek, the other on their genitals. (You can leave your hand there or keep returning if you find it distracting or aren't good at doing two things at once.)

Keep your wrist flexible and cup your hand slightly. Keep your fingers together and spank in a slightly upward motion. This feels better than a downward stroke.

Start soft. Your first spank should be more like a caress than a slap. After you've dispensed it, massage the area for a few seconds and fondle the genitals.

Time the slaps to arrive no more than three to five seconds apart. Cover both cheeks, aiming for the lower (fleshier) part of the cheeks, and start to increase the force. Vary the weight, frequency, and placement of the slaps.

Hold your hand still on the skin for a second or so after a spank. Rub, stroke, or lick the area for a further second, before giving another.

Use an ice cube to cool down the skin after a spank. Then lick or rub it to provide the contrast of hot and cold.

ALL THE WAY

I'm way too jealous to take things this far with my husband, but I can certainly see the attraction. If you're single and desire any or all of the following, why the hell not give it a whirl? (Assuming you practice safe sex, of course; see page 259.) If you're in a relationship that's more about sex than love, and jealousy isn't going to be an issue, again, why not?

But if you are in a happy, monogamous relationship and you're thinking of introducing other warm (hot) bodies into your bed, be aware that you are risking your relationship by doing this. These are activities that need full consent and full approval from both of you before proceeding. If only one is keen and the other isn't, do not go there. You also need to discuss things fully, sleep on it, and discuss again.

SEX CLUBS

Killing Kittens, the Skirt Club—there's a sex party to cater to just about every taste in New York and most other big cities. Guess who they're particularly popular with? Yup—women.

More and more, people are looking outside the traditional monogamous relationship model, and going to a sex party or sex club with your partner is a (relatively) safe first step to experiment with how you'll react to watching each other with others. They're also a safe place to enjoy a girl-on-girl bi-curious encounter, if that piques your interest.

Threesomes, sex parties, and other types of group sex have always been available but not accessible to the general public, let alone participated in by Mr. and Ms. Average (or Ms. and Ms. Average, for that matter). The internet changed all that. Search "sex club" where you live, and if you're close to a city, chances are you'll find something. They range from high class with strict entry criteria to friendlier, casual gatherings. Most have a theme. Choose your poison and take it from there. A lot of clubs are happy for you to go along and watch, rather than participate, but check first.

WOMEN WITH WOMEN

Social psychologist Dr. Justin Lehmiller interviewed 4,175 people for his book *Tell Me What You Want*. It's the largest and most comprehensive survey of Americans' sexual fantasies to date.

Lehmiller found straight women are more open to threesomes with a partner of the same gender and to the idea of an entirely same-sex threesome. "That was the first of many findings in my study that suggested that women may be more erotically flexible than men when it comes to the gender of their partners," he writes. Fifty-nine percent of the women who identified as exclusively straight reported having fantasies about sex with women.

One in four women have had sexual encounters with other women but don't identify as gay or bisexual, according to another study of 24,000 undergraduate students, also in the US. It's increasingly common—much to most men's delight.

Suggest to your male partner that you want to try a same-sex experience, and he will assume this means he's allowed to watch, and while you'll put on a nice show for him, he will think he'll be called on to "properly satisfy" both of you toward the end. Dream on, guys. In reality, if he is allowed to watch, he's completely forgotten as the girls get down to it—often enjoying better sex than they've had with a man.

Another way to indulge a same-sex fantasy is to go to a sex club that caters to women or to a strip club together.

A THREESOME

A study by US sex educator Debby Herbenick and colleagues used a nationally representative sample of over 2,000 American adults aged 18 or over to find out the prevalence and appeal of more than 30 different sexual behaviors. It found one in 10 women and one in five men have had a threesome.

If you're single, not the jealous type, or in a relationship with someone you like but don't love, a threesome can be a highly erotic experience. For lots of loved-up couples, however, it's the worst idea you've ever had.

The obvious, most glaring reason is that couples who love each other usually have a hard time seeing their partners with someone else. No matter how much you've imagined it, you can't really prepare yourself for what it feels like to watch someone else kiss/ touch/cuddle/lick/penetrate your partner.

The fantasy and reality often don't match. Things always go a lot more smoothly in our heads than they do in the bedroom. Most of us cast ourselves in the taking role when we imagine a threesome and get a bit put out when we realize this isn't necessarily the case. Men often feel under such pressure to perform with two women, they can't get an erection. His sexual confidence is shattered to smithereens (What the hell does he tell his friends?) and the ramifications can be dire.

Men often fare worse in general. Lesbians consistently rate highest for the group who are happiest with their sex life. Watching your wife have more—or more intense—orgasms with a woman than she's ever had with you is another nail in the coffin of sexual confidence.

Jealousy in general is an enormous problem—there are three of you in the bed, remember, not two or four, so one person will sometimes feel left out. Do they like the new person more than you? Are they enjoying themselves more with them than they do with you? Is this person better in bed?

Couples who do negotiate it successfully say it's sexually arousing to see someone else make love to their partner. It makes them feel desirable, being with someone who is desired, and that it's instructive to watch other people's sexual techniques. "We wanted to sleep with other people and it seemed more honest to do it in front of each other," said one woman.

Where to indulge? In New York and Los Angeles, there's an app called Feeld for couples and singles who want to meet "open-minded people." Other cities might have similar apps. A sex club is an obvious choice. Or you could hire a sex worker, if you're a couple (though it might be illegal where you live). Swingers clubs are everywhere and another alternative. The worst idea for a first-time threesome is to get drunk and do it with friends. Well, if you value the friendship, that is.

A safer way to get the thrill without the spills is to role-play the idea instead with vibrators, dildos, and a blindfold, or to watch porn together that's based on that theme.

SWINGING

While we're getting rid of sexual stereotypes, you can chuck the one where the man is forcing the woman into swinging. Lehmiller, in his study about sexual fantasies, found 79 percent of men and 62 percent of women had fantasized about being in an open relationship where the partners consent to a set of rules that allow one or both to pursue sex with others. Sixty-six percent of men and 45 percent of women fantasized about swinging.

Swinging is nothing new—it's been around as long as marriage has. If the rumors are to be believed, in the sex-mad seventies, all you had to do was invite all your neighbors over, serve large martinis along with cheese-and-pineapple-on-a-stick canapés (artistically stuck into an orange), and you'd all be pooling your car keys before the first joint got stubbed out. In today's climate, nearly all swingers these days meet at clubs or through websites. Not surprisingly, swinging comes with a hefty "try at your own risk" warning. Most people end up jealous, and it can and does lead to split-ups. On the other hand, lots say it strengthened their relationship rather than ruined it.

Men might be the first to suggest it, but it's not uncommon for women to enjoy it more than they do, once there. Having said that . . .

Don't let anyone force you into swinging. If it's not your thing, it's not your thing. If your partner insists on doing it and you don't want to, rethink the relationship. You both need to be happy and comfortable with the concept and the reality.

Set rules on what's permissible and what's not. Are you going to swing in front of each other or at the same party but privately ("same room" or "separate room")? Are you both going to have full sex with other people or stop at foreplay? Are same-sex encounters allowed? How about group sex?

Some clubs allow you to watch but not participate. If you've never done it before and that's an option, I'd highly advise it. Just being in the environment is enough of a thrill for many couples, and you'll avoid most of the pitfalls by simply watching.

If you try it and like it, you might want to move into an open relationship where you both give each other permission to have other relationships or no-strings sex. Or you might decide you've had your fun but now want to go back to being monogamous.

OPEN MARRIAGE OR POLYAMORY

While most of us admit monogamy isn't perfect but stick with it anyway, some couples decide to open their relationships to outside exploration. Polyamory is romantic love with more than one person. It might mean one or both of you have multiple short- or long-term relationships with other people, as well as each other, with full knowledge and consent.

An open marriage can mean many things, but it usually means that you both give each other approval to have sex with others, within a set of rules agreed on by both of you. If you're not getting your sexual needs met by your partner—they're physically incapable or don't want to have sex anymore for some other reason—and they are happy for you to get them met elsewhere, this is one solution.

HAVE

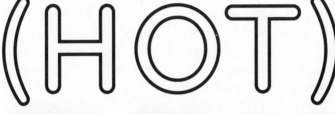

(HOT)
SEX
WITHOUT AN ERECTION

THE LAST FEW CHAPTERS HAVE given you some insight into what's going on in the female brain and body. But what's happening to him? While you're struggling with hot flashes and a dry vagina and/or deciding whether or not to buy a whip, he's trying to come to terms with wobbly erections. And herein lies a huge difference between the sexes.

Most women stoically face the myriad changes happening to their body as they age and simply get on with it. In our eyes, the female equivalent of men having difficulties with erections is not getting "wet." When we were young, we'd think of us being "wet" and him being "hard" as a barometer of how aroused we were. Post-50, most women no longer equate the two because they know they can be as aroused as hell and still not lubricate. It's just what happens when you get older. No big deal, add a bit of lube, and that (particular) problem's solved.

Men don't think this way. And that's putting it mildly. If a man's penis isn't erect, it isn't merely a sign of aging, it's a psychological catastrophe, says New York–based sex therapist Stephen Snyder. Meltdown material.

Here's a handful of the words men use to describe the feeling of not being able to "get it up": Broken. Humiliated. Ashamed. Paranoid. Isolated. Depressed. Emasculated. Suicidal. More than 50,000 men per month visit Frank Talk, which provides support via an anonymous online community, to talk about the devastation of "pushing rope" (trying to penetrate with a semi-erect penis). Many older men would rather not have sex at all than deal with the "disastrous" effects of aging on their penis. "An erection can be the be-all and end-all for some men," says Victoria Lehmann, a UK sex therapist who has decades of experience treating men with erectile dysfunction (ED). "It takes an extraordinary amount of time to convince a man to have any form of sex—oral, hand jobs, kisses, anything—if they aren't getting an erection. Sex, to men, is putting their penis in something. But the reality is there will be unpredictability to his erections as he gets older. Unless he deals with it, sex together is over. You'll both end up either masturbating to porn or not having sex at all."

WHY THE OBSESSION WITH ERECTIONS?

Most of the time, when I interview someone about sex, we have a giggle about something or another. But I learned—fast—not to attempt any type of joke about a penis that refuses to obey its owner. I interviewed many men about sex and aging for this book and not one man under the age of 65 had even remotely come to terms with having erections that weren't "like they were." All were equally resistant to the idea that sex could be good without an erection. "I wouldn't enjoy sex without an erection. Simple as that," says James, a 53-year-old friend of mine who started taking Viagra when his erections became less dependable.

"But you don't *need* an erect penis to have a great time in bed," I counter, trotting out a line I estimate I've used about 5,000 times in my career. "That's from the woman's perspective," he says. "She doesn't need a man to be erect to get pleasure from oral sex, for instance. But a man needs an erection in order to be aroused while giving her oral sex. Even if you know sex isn't going to include penetration, an erection is necessary. It's not a macho thing, it's a physical thing. The blood has to pump into the penis for men to feel any desire at all."

Which leaves a lot of men over 50 stuck between a rock and a (not so) hard place, given firm, reliable erections are less and less likely as he ages.

Even if they do achieve an erection, anxiety over losing it ruins sex for many men. In his book *Love Worth Making*, Snyder writes, "Making love while worrying about staying hard is a bit like trying to enjoy a movie while worrying about whether the projector is going to work. You're not going to be able to enjoy the movie very much. After a while, you're not going to want to go back to that theatre either. Worrying about erections is probably the most common reason men avoid sex. Having an erection is no guarantee that he'll enjoy himself. But if he doesn't have one, there's not much chance he'll remember the experience fondly."

Understanding just how devastated men feel when their penis stops performing like it used to is paramount to enjoying *any* sex post-50, let alone decent sex. Take a moment to let that really sink in. Men. Are. Terrified. Of. A. Penis. That. Doesn't. Work.

Why are men so anxious about sex?

Male anxiety is on the rise, and yes, it does have to do with porn and the messages it sends men. In porn, men get instant erections just by looking at something sexy and have penises that are as thick and hard as their wrist. But "it's the double punch of porn and Viagra that's so persuasive—and dangerous," says US sex therapist Ian Kerner in his book *He Comes Next*.

Kerner believes male anxiety is on the rise because the pharmaceutical industry is targeting men—young and old—with erectile stimulants (like Viagra) and bombarding them with marketing messages that reinforce a "penis-focused, intercourse-based vision of sex that preys on performance anxiety and breeds spectatoring." *Spectatoring* is when a person mentally watches themself having sex, rather than being in the moment. Some therapists believe it's the primary cause of most sexual dysfunction in men.

Before drugs like Viagra, Kerner writes, couples dealt with the issue of ED through intimacy-building exercises, erotic creativity, and communication. "Men were significantly more likely to address ED holistically. Now, a little blue pill solves the problem. But it does so in a way that's purely physiological. Before, men were encouraged to think beyond their penises and make love with more than just their penises. The irony is that while these desire-building activities didn't always lead to consistent erections, they did often result in greater intimacy, stronger relationships, increased desire, and yes, more female orgasms."

Viagra may not be the "lifesaver" men think it is

A lot of people who know their stuff sexually believe the use of Viagra is reinforcing bad habits and encouraging bad sex. For starters, hard erections aren't necessarily what women want. "The drug companies focus on men. They aren't asking the 30 million women who will be on the receiving end of those erections," Kerner says.

In a sense, we're working against nature using PDE5 medications (like Viagra). As a woman's vaginal lining gets thinner and she becomes more sensitive, his erection gets softer. The two work well together. What often doesn't work is a steel-hard erection with an older vagina. He suddenly has the erection of a young man and is, understandably, overjoyed about it. His wife may not be; it's going to hurt. Some men are so determined to use their new youthful erections that if their wife refuses to have intercourse, they go outside the relationship to test drive.

Victoria Lehmann believes Viagra is useful. "It can be easier to slip in a hard penis than stuff in a soft one," she says pragmatically.

"But it has to be spoken about, you must use lube, and test drive the vagina: massage inside first, to make sure she's ready."

Snyder's view on Viagra and other PDE5-inhibitor medications is that it can be "an act of mercy" for the man to take them. "They don't always work—especially if his erection problems are more advanced, or their emotional problems are more serious." But, for many couples, medication just makes it easier to get things going in an erotic direction. "Maybe in the future, we'll have evolved to where middle-aged men can enjoy lovemaking without having to worry about their erections. But I'm not holding my breath." And wait—there's more. A lot of men are also convinced getting an erection is "proof " of their desire for their partner and it's insulting to her when they don't have one. Their relationship is at risk, as well as their sex life. The poor bastards! Is it any wonder a semi-erect or flaccid penis scares the hell out of men?

Is an erect penis "evidence" of desire?

Here's what women said when I asked them if they felt offended when their partner couldn't get an erection.

"I never took it personally."

"He's nearly 60, of course he's going to have problems. It's nothing to do with me."

"Maybe a little disappointed but never offended."

"I'm overjoyed. I'd prefer sex without intercourse these days—no soreness afterward and no UTI."

"I'm secure in myself. I don't relate my attractiveness to his erection difficulties."

Younger women might question how "sexy" they are when men's penises don't bound eagerly to their tummies the second they undress, but most older women are far too realistic and grounded to worry.

I'm back interviewing James, two glasses of wine in, and tell him the reactions I got when I asked women if they think no erection equals no desire for them. He lifts his eyebrows and looks surprised—and unconvinced. "Say your wife can't tolerate penetration anymore and it's never going to be in the cards, would getting an erection be important then?" I ask. Come on, I've got you with this one!

"It's not about whether you'll use it to penetrate," he says, in a you-just-don't-get-this-do-you exasperated tone. "An erection is a man's physical manifestation of his desire for a woman. It makes her feel desired and that's really important for her to know that he finds her sexually attractive."

He's right that women need to feel desired. What he's not getting is that we don't need the "evidence" of an erect penis to know if a man is turned on by us or not. We see desire in the way our partner looks at us, a hooding of the eyes, a swelling of the mouth, the way he touches us and licks us.

Gay men, lesbians, and other LGBTQIA people don't seem to be as hung up on the whole erection thing as straight people are. "Most straight couples see intercourse as the only really 'grown-up' way to have sex, and they feel like failures if for whatever reason intercourse isn't working for them," Snyder believes. For people with different sexual orientations, penile penetration seems very much a take-it-or-leave-it thing rather than the main event. Sensible, if you ask me.

WHAT CAUSES ERECTION PROBLEMS

Wondrous and impressive as it is, an erection is simply a penis that's full of blood. An erection happens when blood flows into the two chambers inside the penis, making it hard. If he's having erection problems, issues with blood flow are often to blame.

Unfortunately for men, there's rather a lot of things than can affect it. Medical conditions like diabetes, heart disease, and high blood pressure are culprits, as is obesity. Low testosterone levels affect libido and erection quality. If your man has an unhealthy lifestyle—smokes, drinks heavily, doesn't exercise, eats food high in saturated fat, and doesn't get enough sleep—I have zero doubt he has erection problems if he's over 50.

Add some anxiety and stress into the mix and things worsen. If he's stressed, you're having relationship issues, he's worried about work, exhausted, depressed, or traumatized by something, this will all affect how his penis performs. Any type of anxiety triggers the fight-or-flight reflex that sends blood away from the penis (always bad news) to the limbs for self-defense or escape.

Sometimes, erection problems are caused when the penis can't trap blood during an erection, something that can happen at any age. Certain diseases, injury, or surgery in the pelvic area can harm nerves to the penis, and some cancer treatments near the pelvis can affect its functionality. Prostate, colorectal, or bladder cancer often leaves men with ED. Peyronie's disease—which causes penises to bend—can also have an effect. Benign prostatic hyperplasia (BPH) is a noncancerous enlargement of the prostate gland that can also cause urinary problems and difficulties with erections.

Because erection problems are also symptoms of other, more serious health issues, it's extremely important that any man who notices a change sees a doctor.

The difference between aging erections and ED

It's estimated that ED affects over half of all men aged between 50 and 70. Most middle-age erection changes, however, are not ED but "erection dissatisfaction." This means it takes longer for him to get an erection, they're less firm and dependable, and he needs manual or oral stimulation to get hard. This isn't dysfunction, it's a normal and inevitable consequence of aging.

A better definition for "true" ED is not being able to get an erection during extended masturbation, or when he's not under the influence of alcohol or other erection-impairing drugs (recreational and some prescription drugs like antidepressants or opiates, which can significantly contribute to ED). A man who fails to have an erection more than 50 percent of the time would also probably get the clinical diagnosis of ED. For the sake of simplicity, I'll refer to both erection dissatisfaction and erectile dysfunction as ED, but it can be reassuring for men to know the difference.

One major problem with ED is that men of all ages can literally think themselves into having it: it happens once, they're anxious the next time, so it happens again. Before long, a few "failed" attempts at intercourse have created a cycle of ongoing ED. The more he worries about it, the more likely it is to happen the next time.

How to tell whether the cause is physical or psychological? One easy way is to establish whether he gets an erection during sleep, when he's not plagued by anxiety. The traditional way to test this was to attach a ring of postage stamps around the base of his penis before going to bed and check to see if it was broken when he woke up. If it was, he'd had a sleep erection and the problem wasn't physical. Needless to say, this method was fraught with problems (they'd fall off, he'd forget they were there when he went for a pee . . .). Besides, who has loads of stamps hanging around these days?

A simpler way to figure it out is to establish whether he wakes up with an early-morning erection or achieves one when he's masturbating on his own. If he can, the cause probably isn't physical. If the answer is no, and no, it probably is. (Don't be offended, by the way, if you find out he can get erect when you aren't around. It simply means there's less anxiety.)

The more clues you have about what's causing his erection problems the better: it helps determine how you try to solve the problem, if you see it as one. The fact is, he doesn't need an erection to orgasm. Different nerves govern erection and orgasm. Semi-erect or flaccid penises can produce orgasms just as intense as those he had with a rock-solid hard-on.

HOW TO TALK TO HIM ABOUT ERECTION PROBLEMS

It can be terrifying talking about sex issues. The good news is, once you get past those first few awkward minutes, most couples find it's much easier than they thought—and an incredible relief to finally get it out in the open.

Choose a time when you're getting along well and a place where you can most comfortably chat. It might be over a drink at the end of day or while cooking dinner together. Try to make sure there are no interruptions. Bring up the subject by simply saying, "Have you noticed we're not having sex as much lately? I miss it. Why do you think that is? Shall we talk about it?"

See it from his side. If he's not very good at expressing emotion, sex was probably how he expressed love for you. If you're not having it, he worries about the impact that's having. He may be worried you'll stop loving him, find sex elsewhere, or are laughing at him behind his back. The more anxious he feels, the worse the problem gets. He may be avoiding sex with you and having solo sex instead. This doesn't mean he doesn't desire or love you; he's just too embarrassed to let you see what's happening.

Write down what you'd like to say, so you can word it properly. Use "I" not "you" when you do. ("I worry you don't find me attractive when you don't want sex" rather than "You make me feel unattractive when you don't want sex.") Say it out loud solo. How would you react if you heard that? Is it sensitively and tactfully worded?

Tell him you love him, miss sex with him, and want to talk about why you're both not having it anymore. He may react angrily or defensively, but stay calm. Tell him you don't automatically feel like sex all the time, and perhaps it's the same for him. Tell him you read that half of all men over 40 get erection problems at some stage, and ask if that's happening to him and that's why he's avoiding sex.

Constantly reassure him that it happens to everyone, and is normal and fixable. Let him know you don't need him to get an erection to enjoy sex, to take the pressure off. But do encourage him to see his doctor because it can mean other health issues. Offer to go with him.

Focus on solutions, rather than the problem. Read this chapter through together and use it as a talking point.

If he refuses to talk, drop it and say, "I'm here if you'd like to talk to me later." Try again in a few days. Encourage even small attempts from him to open up. Nearly all men say they feel so much better once they've talked with their partners and are ready to find a solution.

TREATMENTS FOR ED

Most men find it shaming to seek help for ED. Men are supposed to always want sex and always be ready for it. It's emasculating when this doesn't happen, which is incredibly sad since there are many treatments for ED and lots that he can do to drastically improve erection quality. Such as . . .

A change of lifestyle. Exercise keeps the blood flowing and his arteries producing nitric oxide, which is an important molecule for blood-vessel health. Nitric oxide is produced by the linings of the blood vessels (endothelium) as the blood flow increases, helping to sustain an erection and the nerve endings innervating the penis.

A poor diet contributes to heart disease, high cholesterol, and arterial plaque—all inhibit blood flow to the penis. If he stops smoking, loses weight, and cuts back on alcohol, his erections should improve; getting stress under control is another factor. Anxiety is a libido flattener and antidepressants further depress desire.

Testosterone supplements. He should ask his doctor to test his levels. If they're low, they'll usually recommend a testosterone gel (or similar) that can dramatically increase libido within weeks. It can have an effect on erection quality as well.

Counseling. If his ED is psychological—caused by stress, depression, or anxiety—"talk" therapy can be highly effective. Seeing a therapist either individually or as a couple can also help other treatments work more effectively.

Oral drugs (Viagra, Levitra, Cialis, and Stendra or Spedra [avanafil], which contain PDE5 inhibitors). Medications like Viagra relax the blood vessels that supply blood to the penis, so blood can flow into it freely to create an erection. They work on about two-thirds of men, but for Viagra (the most popular), 48 percent of men report suffering at least one side effect.

Viagra works between 30 minutes and an hour after taking a tablet and works best when taken on an empty stomach. The effects last for four to six hours. Levitra also lasts around four to six hours, but it's less affected by food or alcohol—helpful if you plan on eating or drinking before sex. Cialis lasts much longer than Viagra or Levitra (up to 36 hours), so it's more conducive to spontaneous sex. The downside is the possible side effects last longer, too. Cialis isn't affected by food, but alcohol does reduce the effects. Stendra and Spedra are the newest boys on the block and can work in 15 minutes. Before taking any of these drugs, you must check with your doctor whether they react negatively with other medication you're taking, plus get a general health check.

Which is right for your partner? He won't know the answer to that unless he tries them all. Visit your doctor and get a prescription. Don't even think about buying on the internet from a site you don't know. If you don't know where you're buying the drugs from, you don't know what's in them, and they put pretty dangerous stuff in some of them (rat poison, for one).

The side effects of all the oral drugs are similar: headaches, facial flushing (or "having a big red head," as one man described it to me, "which is so noticeable, people comment"), feeling sleepy afterward, nasal congestion, and aching muscles.

Vacuum or penis pumps. These are airtight plastic cylinders that slip over the penis and pump out the air, which draws blood into the penile chambers to produce an erection. He can then use a penis ring (or cock ring), which sits at the base of the penis, to trap the blood inside. The Urology Care Foundation (US) says, with training, about 75 out of 100 men can get a working erection using this method (though lots of couples find it intrusive).

Injectable medicines. Alprostadil injections can be used by men who can't take oral drugs or find they don't work. The idea of injecting their penis sends most men skedaddling, but those who've done it say it's almost painless, if expensive. With training, the success rate is as high as 85 percent with this treatment.

Penile implants. These work well if the cause of the ED is physical. There are two types. Semi-rigid rods make the penis firm enough for penetration but flexible enough to conceal an erection while clothed. They're permanent and his erection doesn't alter: it's permanently in this state. Inflatable implants involve pressing a pump (usually in the scrotum or lower abdomen) to fill the implants on demand. He's got more control and the erections are more natural.

HOW WOMEN FEEL ABOUT VIAGRA

Men might be besotted with the little blue pill, but women's reactions are mixed. "It's made sex even more of an effort," said one 59-year-old woman. "Our entire day now gets planned around it. We can't go out for a boozy lunch like we used to before sex, because Viagra doesn't work as well if he drinks too much. We can't enjoy a nice meal because it doesn't work on a full stomach. Afterward, he feels really tired and not up for doing anything and his face is bright red, so he feels embarrassed going out. All this just so he gets erect for about 20 minutes! I'd rather enjoy the day and have sex without an erection."

Because lots of men see Viagra as the one and only solution, if it doesn't work for them, they give up on sex entirely, not bothering to try other methods. "My partner needs Viagra to perform but he gets dreadful headaches from them," one woman told me. "He won't try any of the other drugs because his doctor told him they don't work as well. He's totally unwilling to explore any other alternative solution because, in his eyes, if Viagra won't work, nothing will. We used to have sex once or twice a year, now it's never. He's not affectionate because he's worried it will lead to sex. At 53, I still want to be sexual. I won't look elsewhere but I'm sad it's come to this, and I wonder, if Viagra wasn't invented, if he'd have dealt with it a whole lot better."

Many (many) women talked about how Viagra made their partner's erections too hard and said they felt enormous pressure to have penetrative sex even when it hurt.

But others say Viagra saved their sex life. The plain cold reality is lots of men won't consider having sex without an erection, and Viagra helps between 60 and 70 percent of men achieve this. "The minute he couldn't get an erection, his whole attitude to sex changed," said one woman. "It became 'What's the point?' No thought to whether I was ready to give up sex! This lasted for two years. Then one day, out of the blue, he starts kissing me passionately and I could feel he had an erection. I asked him if it was from Viagra, and he told me not to 'spoil it' by asking. So, I don't. I'm just grateful it's brought him back to bed."

Other comments included: "It makes him relax." "It gives him confidence." "It makes him feel like him again. Like when he was young." Each person is different, each couple is different. In my experience, most couples try a drug like Viagra as their first solution and explore other methods after that. The temptation to take a pill and all could be fixed is too strong to resist.

HOW TO HAVE GREAT SEX WITHOUT HIS PENIS BEING THE STAR

It's ironic that the reason older people often report better sex lives than younger people is because age often brings erectile dysfunction to men. If men can learn to relax into sex that isn't intercourse focused, they learn to enjoy foreplay. Because they take longer to get aroused—which may or may not produce an erection—they spend more time on pleasuring us, making for better sex all around. Good for both of you, but particularly for women because we orgasm from stimulation of the clitoris, not through penetration.

I'm sure all of you know by now, but it's worth repeating that about 70 to 80 percent of women don't orgasm from penetration alone. Intercourse is often the least-interesting part of sex for women. It might freak the hell out of men, but if your partner does make peace with erection issues, it's nearly always good news for older women.

Here's how to make the most out of nonpenetrative sex.

Help him accept what's happening. Crack this and the rest is easy. If you've dutifully read this chapter from the start, you'll have gotten the message, loud and clear, about how significant getting hard is to him. Don't just approach the topic with kid gloves; imagine you're holding a just-hatched chick in the palm of your hand.

There's a section on how to broach the topic on page 140. Ideally, you'd get to the point where he feels comfortable enough to talk about the problem with you, and you decide together how you're going to tackle it.

The more involved you are in this process, the less impact it will have on your sex life. Try not to get upset or frustrated if he refuses to talk or, in your opinion, is overreacting to something that's quite normal. For lots of men, dealing with erection problems is one of the hardest things they've done. I can see your raised eyebrow from here, reading that statement (and I agree with you). But it doesn't matter if you think that's pathetic, it's how he views it that's crucial here.

Don't let him avoid sex and hide. The average man takes two to three years before seeing a doctor about a sex problem.

Most don't talk to their partner either. They think if they don't talk about it and avoid sex for a while, the problem will "sort itself out." It won't.

Never call him impotent. Sex therapist Esther Perel hates the word. "It's ugly," she says in her *Where Should We Begin?* podcasts. "I hate labels. Language shapes the experience. If you say to a man, 'You're impotent,' you define him by it. You guarantee that is what he will be from now on. It's a horrible word. Don't say it out loud."

Sex isn't just about the genitals. "Impotence doesn't define someone," Perel continues. "We make love with our whole body, not just our genitals. A good thing, too, because we can't rely on them." Happily, you can rely on your hands, skin, mouth, voice, smile, eyes: those things don't change. "If you let an erection be the focus of sex, you are missing the point. It's not about the penis. It's about emotion, connection, skin, touching, talking, playing," she says.

Let him know you can take care of yourself. If he knows you can climax through other means—a vibrator, him using his tongue or his fingers—the pressure for getting erect lessens.

Stop trying to be young. Change the focus. It's not about penetration, erections, or orgasms anymore. Stop pining over the sex you used to have. This is new, different, and exciting.

Think slow and lazy. Take your time. Get naked. Have lots of deep kissing. Lie back in each other's arms and pleasure yourself, either using your hands or a sex toy while they watch. Or let them do it. Remember, sex doesn't have to include an orgasm for each of you—or any orgasms at all. Take the pressure off.

Take a break from intercourse. "Simply taking a break from the goal of achieving intercourse can help with a substantial number of sex problems," Snyder says.

Give sexual compliments. How much you love a certain part of their body. The way their skin feels. How they make you feel. How good they are at what they're doing. Feeling loved, accepted, and wanted sexually is a big part of sexual self-esteem for men.

Focus on what's going right, not what's going wrong. Glass half full, not half empty. There's lots to love about sex when you're older. Start appreciating what you do have.

THE PROSTATE: HITTING THE "P" SPOT

The anus is packed with nerve endings and is a hot spot for both sexes but particularly for men because it's the home of the prostate gland (also known as the male G-spot).

Gay men discovered how pleasurable prostate massage could be ages ago. Now prostate-stimulating toys are one of the fastest-growing markets in sex toys. Not only is it something new to try, but stimulating his P spot can also improve the firmness and quality of his erections. Here's how.

- Pick your time. Many a lover's hand has been brushed aside while tentatively exploring, never to return again, not because their partner wasn't interested but because they were worried the three-course gassy dinner they've just polished off might make the experience, well, use your imagination.

- Add lube to your finger or partner's anus and start by rubbing your fingertip gently around the rim until the muscles relax. Use the finger you point with to begin with, inserting it a tiny way, then waiting for the rectum to get used to the sensation. (Nails short and trimmed, please.)

- Keep inserting it, a little at a time, and once it's all in there, hold it still. The rectum is used to things coming out, not going in, and even if this new intruder is welcome, it still takes time to get used to it.

- The prostate feels like a ripe plum and you'll find it about 2 inches inside. It's easier to find in older men because the gland gets larger with age.

- Try making a beckoning, "come here" motion with your finger or make small circles. Don't thrust in and out, like you might while pushing a finger inside the vagina. Try tapping. Keep the pressure firm but not hard.

- Don't worry if he loses his erection during anal stimulation, says Ian Kerner in *He Comes Next*. "Some men, for a combination of psychological and physiological reasons, cannot maintain a full erection when penetrated." It doesn't mean you're not doing it right.

- Add some oral sex or hand action for the best effect.

- He liked it? Invest in one of the many new sex toys specifically designed to massage his prostate (see page 173).

IF YOU DO WANT TO TRY FOR AN ERECTION

You're happy if he doesn't achieve one but no harm in trying? Here are some things that will up the chances of an erection happening. But all come with this proviso: play, don't pressure. Look or act desperate for any of this to "work" and you're in for a horrible, stressful experience. Forget any end goal. Instead, simply enjoy trying new things for their own sake and go wherever it takes you.

If you are using a drug like Viagra

- Make sure he takes it on an empty stomach. For this reason, it can work better if you have sex in the morning rather than at night.

- He can reduce anxiety by having a hot shower before sex, breathing deeply during it, and focusing on the sensations he's feeling rather than what his penis is up to.

- The refractory period—the time between ejaculation and orgasm and his next erection—gets longer as he gets older. If you know you'll be having sex that night, it's better if he doesn't masturbate for at least a day beforehand.

- Plan when you'll have sex. That way he can manage the medication. A lot of older men say they feel more comfortable knowing when sex will happen.

- Viagra doesn't cause an instant erection. He still needs firm stimulation for an erection to happen.

- Don't forget yourself, as well! Make sure he understands you need plenty of warm-up before he penetrates or it will hurt. Use bucket loads of good-quality lube and get him to penetrate slowly, stopping every inch to let you relax around him before continuing.

- If his Viagra-induced erection hurts too much for you to enjoy sex, tell him. You can both enjoy his erection without having to have intercourse, and simply having an erection during sex is great news for men. Even if they don't put it inside anything.

- Finally, don't expect miracles. It can take a little time for the medication to build up in his system.

No Viagra required

- Consider using a strap-on. He can't take the pills or you both aren't interested in him taking them? Here's an easy way to have an erection that never lets you down: buy a strap-on dildo with a harness. (See page 175 if you need details or convincing.)

- Whatever you do, use lube. Post-50, lube is as essential to sex as oxygen is for breathing.

- Build desire. Don't grab straight for his penis and start pumping. Excite his eyes by watching porn together or a sexy movie. Or let him watch you touch yourself. Kiss his neck. Cup his testicles. Grasp his penis and stretch the skin toward the scrotum to increase sensitivity. Do this a few times. Squeeze his nipples. Make eye contact. Tell him what you're going to do or how turned on it makes you feel. If he keeps grabbing your hand and wanting you to go straight to pumping, tie his wrists together. Run your hand up his penis, hold it, and squeeze. Then use your fingers to squeeze up and down the shaft.

- Now you can use firmer stimulation. Older men generally like quite vigorous stimulation. Get him to show you what technique he uses when he masturbates and put your hand on top of his to get a feel for how he uses his hand. Most important: watch where and how he first grips his penis and replicate it. It makes all the difference. (There are more tips on how to give good hand on page 46.)

- Take your time. Men need more and longer direct stimulation to achieve an erection or to become aroused when they're older. Make sure you're comfortable and settle in, making it clear to him that he can relax, lie back, and simply enjoy what you're doing.

- Slip on a "stroker." More about these ingenious inventions in chapter 2. They're soft tubes or sleeves, usually made of silicone, that you slide over the penis (add lube first), then slide up and down using your hand. Strokers instantly transform a ho-hum hand job into the best he's ever had because they intensify sensation.

- Try a penis ring. They sit at the base of his penis to trap the blood inside, retaining an erection for longer. More on how to use these on page 144.

- Press other hot spots simultaneously. Double stimulation is effective. While you're working on his penis, put your hand on his lower belly and rub slowly but firmly to stimulate his inner penis. Or hold your hand in an L-shape on its side and position it between his legs, then push up firmly. This provides strong pressure on the perineum and base of his testicles.

- Add some anal stimulation. Put a well-lubed finger inside his anus (see "The Prostate: Hitting the 'P' Spot," page 149), or insert a butt plug and leave it there while you stimulate him elsewhere. Vibrating prostate stimulators (see page 149) have revived many an older man's interest in sex.

- Penises make great masturbatory tools. Sit astride him, add lube, then "wrap" your labia around the shaft of his penis—it doesn't matter whether he's hard or soft—and grind against it. Lots of women can orgasm this way. Or use the oh-so-soft head to masturbate your clitoris.

- Put it between your breasts, after adding lots of lube, and get him to thrust in between.

- Use dildos. Take the pressure off both of you by investing in some dildos (glass dildos are both beautiful and versatile) and/or insertable vibrators so you aren't reliant on his erection. Great for role-playing, too.

- Stop chasing erections and start having fun. Try spanking each other. Have long, erotic oral sex sessions where you immerse yourselves in each other's bodies. Give massages, play games.

- Try doggy style if/when you're ready to be penetrated, but spread your legs extra wide. If he loses his erection, he can pull out to stroke himself, hold his finger on the underside of the penis, acting like a splint, or grasp hard at the base for maximum control.

SEX AFTER PROSTATE CANCER

As with any disease, prostate cancer doesn't just affect the patient. It can have a profound effect on a couple's sex life and relationship. Things have improved, though—dramatically.

There was a time when urologists would discuss every side effect except sexual function, but that's all changed. Even before any definite treatment plan for the prostate cancer is agreed upon, part of the discussion usually includes informing the patient, often with their partner present, exactly what the couple will be dealing with postsurgery.

This includes frank discussion, where appropriate, about erectile dysfunction (ED). Psychosexual counseling is usually available as part of rehabilitation, and lots of patients benefit from this, sometimes starting before any treatment even begins.

There are things he can do to speed up recovery. Some surgeons recommend a nightly low dose of Viagra (or similar) to keep the penis oxygenated during sleep. Gentle stretching and massage helps, as does using a penis pump that draws blood into the penis and out again. Maintaining a healthy blood flow to the penis is essential. Pelvic-floor exercises, squeezing and releasing the same muscle he uses to stop the flow of urine, are also a good idea. Also remember there are alternative PDE5 inhibitors if the one that's prescribed doesn't agree with him. Be patient; it can take up to three years for stretched nerves, unavoidable during surgery, to recover.

Emotionally, it can be difficult. Incontinence can affect his quality of life, ED is common, and some men lose length in their penis. It's not unusual for men to stop having sex after prostate surgery out of embarrassment and shame. His body image suffers and lots of men say they feel less attractive. Affection can disappear along with sex: what happens if he cuddles you, you expect more, and he can't deliver? Meanwhile, you're nervous about suggesting sex, in case he's not ready for it, which some men interpret as you not wanting to have sex with a man whose penis isn't what it was.

Each man's experience is highly individual and reflects their personality and level of coping skills. As always, couples who talk openly with each other about what's going on survive the journey and negotiate their way to a new style of sex that's gentler and less penetration focused, but also more loving and intimate. Communication is key, and you'll find lots of information about how to broach sensitive topics like ED on page 140.

Here's what some women told me about their experience with partners who've had prostate surgery:

- "When my husband was first diagnosed with prostate cancer and we knew he had to have surgery, our doctor recommended that we go away for a week and have as much sex as we could. At the time we were only just coping emotionally and that idea didn't really appeal to us. Now, when I think about it, we should have taken the doctor's advice!"

- "He's bitter about it. He's always ridiculing himself and pretty much thinks life is over now that he's not the owner of a big, hard penis. I try to be sympathetic, but I find it irritating and a bit pathetic. Women don't behave like that after a hysterectomy."

- "He grieved afterward. Especially when he realized the impotence wasn't temporary and that sensation was greatly reduced. But, over a period of years, he learned to enjoy sex again by paying more attention to things like kissing, oral sex, and stroking. We're fine now."

- "My partner's cancer was very aggressive, and that gives you a huge reality check. His life is way, way more important to us than our sex life. That is still the case. I think we are both very happy for what we have considering what he went through."

- "Once I realized he wasn't going to die, I was secretly quite pleased. Penetration had hurt for ages, and I'd been pretending to like sex when actually I'd come to dread it. The thought of never having to have intercourse again makes me happy, not sad."

- "Sure, his erection isn't like it used to be, but we aren't complaining. But I know it's not the same for him and that makes me feel sad. His orgasms are far less intense. He said it's like the difference between a deep, passionate kiss and a butterfly kiss. I sometimes feel hurt that he doesn't enjoy it as much. Like I should be sexy enough to make it as good as it was. But obviously I know it's nothing to do with me and everything to do with the side effects of the operation."

- "Maybe if we'd been younger, we wouldn't have coped so well. Being our ages (we're both over 60) and having been married for 40 years, there is so much love and respect, and I don't feel like I am missing out on anything."

WHY

SEX TOYS

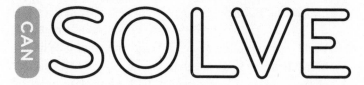

CAN SOLVE

MOST OF

YOUR PROBLEMS

THE WORLD DIVIDES US INTO those who've used sex toys and those who haven't. I discovered vibrators—my big sister's "back massager," hidden in the back of a cupboard—when I was 15. It was my first orgasm and an eye-opening, sheet-clutching, life-changing experience. (Even if the first thing I did afterward was check I hadn't wet myself. Why don't they teach you this stuff at school?)

Like most women who've used a vibrator, I've never looked back. When my time is over and I'm at the pearly gates, I'll be having a good look to see if there are any vibrators up there. If not, I'm heading in the other direction; a sex life that doesn't include sex toys is unthinkable to me.

Yet there's a whole generation of women in their forties, fifties, and over who missed the vibrator revolution and never caught up. A recent UK survey of 2,000 women over 40 found just over one-quarter owned a vibrator and 68 percent had no sex toys whatsoever. Only 30 percent said sex toys would play a useful role in couple's sex. This is in stark contrast to younger women: a quarter of those now own at least three.

Apathy rather than enthusiasm cropped up in my post-50 research as well. These were the answers when I asked the question "Do you use sex toys?":

"I don't bother with things like that."

"My husband brought something home once, but I don't think we ever used it. Don't know what all the fuss is about."

"I never really got the whole vibrator thing. I've got a husband, why would I want one?"

The women who answered "no" to the question also rated their sex-life satisfaction as low. This doesn't surprise me in the slightest. If you are a woman over 50 who doesn't own a vibrator, buying and using one will almost certainly guarantee you are more sexually satisfied than you are now. About half of all women in the US have used a vibrator and these women are more likely to report better arousal, desire, and orgasm.

If you've never had an orgasm, your best possible chance is with a vibrator. If you've never had an orgasm during penetration, it's a vibrator that will get you there. If you've never had an orgasm with your partner, the best possible way is to invite your vibrator into bed with the two of you. If you want to orgasm more quickly, a vibrator is your best bet. For most women, nothing—not even damn fine oral sex—can bring us to orgasm more easily and effectively than vibration.

HERE'S WHAT ELSE OWNING A SEX TOY WILL DO FOR YOU

As your body changes and medical conditions start appearing, so do sex problems. But for every problem, there's a solution—and that solution is often a sex toy. If you used to masturbate using your fingers, that might not be possible if your wrists aren't strong or you have arthritic fingers. Today's lightweight vibrators solve that issue with the press of a button.

If you're single or not having sex with your partner, sex toys keep everything in good working order and you sexually satisfied. Masturbating regularly has enormous physical and emotional benefits. For a start, orgasms reduce anxiety and stop us getting depressed. "It truly is a case of 'use it or lose it' with our genitals," says sex therapist Victoria Lehmann. "If you're not having regular sex, you need to keep your genitals responsive by massaging the vaginal wall with a sex toy. Use them on the clitoris to bring yourself to orgasm to give your pelvic floor muscles a workout. It's not going to be very comfortable when you do have intercourse again otherwise."

And wait, there's more

Even if you're in a relationship and having sex with a partner, sex toys are indispensable. If you're going through a low or no-sex stage, they maintain the sexual stimulation that increases blood flow to help counter dryness and decreased elasticity, which makes us feel sore. If you're not having regular sex with your partner, have it with yourself.

Most women masturbate quickly and reliably on their own with a vibrator. It's much harder to orgasm with a partner because there's another element: a real person. Someone you need to think about and worry about. Your vibrator won't be offended if you turn it up or down or move it this way or that. Solo sex is selfish sex—the best kind—which is why older women often have it more often than they have sex with their partner. It doesn't matter how you have them: the bottom line is the more orgasms the better when you age.

Sex toys provide specific and controllable stimulation—you can turn them up or down depending on what you need—unlike fingers, tongues, and penises. Very handy, if you're finding it harder to climax. They're even more useful to speed up arousal; vibration quickly gets blood flowing to our hot spots, which is what makes us feel aroused.

If his erections aren't hard enough, or it takes either of you too long to orgasm, they're a guaranteed way to tip you over the edge. Just knowing there's a fail-safe way to give you an orgasm that has nothing to do with his penis performing can make sex more enjoyable for both of you.

Equally as important, sex toys introduce variety and are a safe, inexpensive, effortless way of doing it. There is a bewildering array of products out there. Today's vibrators don't just vibrate, they rotate, penetrate, swirl, lick, and seek out parts our parents didn't know existed. They come disguised as bedside lamps, flashlights, lipstick, mobile phones, iPods, and rubber duckies. There are toys for our mouths, bottoms, breasts, nipples, penises, perineums, vaginas, clitorises, and urethras. There are vibrators so small you can lose them in your handbag, and so big they look like a rolling pin.

Sex toys now are better because they're designed by women

One of them is me. I have been a consultant for several companies over the years and currently have two product lines—Supersex and Edge—with a company called Lovehoney that operates in Australia, the US, the UK, and some European countries. I have around 50 products in total and a funny story to go with nearly all of them. (Sadly, another book, another time; there's too much else I have to tell you for this one!) Some of them are specifically designed with older women in mind; if you want to check them out, they are the "Soft Feel" products and you'll find them on my website, traceycox.com.

Lots of sex-toy retailers now use female designers. Compare the old, hard, black rattlers with today's sophisticated, velvet-smooth sex toys and you just know women have got their hands on them.

CHOOSING THE RIGHT SEX TOY FOR YOU

Where are you going to use it?

What body part do you want to stimulate? The clitoris, vagina, nipples, G-spot? Do you want to use it solo or with your partner?

Do you want to use it for penetration or just clitoral stimulation? Vaginal tissue gets more delicate as we age, so even if you were a fan of penetration, you might not be now. If you aren't, don't pay for more toy than you use. Lots of women are brainwashed to think "rabbit" vibes—the world's most famous vibrator—are the best. They are great, if you want to insert the shaft and use the ears on the clitoris. But if the vibrating "ears" are the only thing you're using, the most expensive part of the toy is wasted.

HOW TO MASTURBATE

Everyone knows how to masturbate, right? You'd be surprised. I'm betting there are more than a few of you reading this who have never explored your own body. If that's you, you'll find this useful: a guide to the three most popular methods women use to masturbate.

Usually, we'll watch porn or erotica, read a sexy book, or run a raunchy fantasy or past sexual experience through our heads while enjoying a solo sex session. If you're on medication or suffer from ailments, also think about what time of the day you feel at your best and (obviously) when you're least likely to be interrupted.

You'll notice none of these techniques include putting anything inside the vagina. That's because 80 to 90 percent of women don't use penetration when they masturbate. If you'd like to, go right ahead (a "rabbit" vibe is best for you, if that's your thing).

WITH A VIBRATOR

Obviously, all vibrators are different, so read the instructions first. (If there aren't any included, you'll usually find them online, along with a video in lots of cases, if you look up the brand.) The standard technique is to press it firmly against the closed labia (lips of the vagina) and hold it there, varying the pressure, until you orgasm. Try doing it standing up, sitting with legs apart, or lying down. Another technique is to stand with your legs apart, hold the vibrator still in front of your genitals and move backward and forward, grinding against it. Moving it in a circular motion is also popular, as well as kneeling on the floor and squatting over it.

Adjust the intensity by putting your hand over the vibe to absorb the vibration, removing it when you want it stronger again. Try angling it so it's jutting into the side of the clitoris with the outer labia as a buffer. Or put a soft T-shirt between it and you. You can also try holding your middle fingers over your clitoris and putting the vibrator on top.

USING YOUR FINGERS

If you don't want to use a sex toy, don't have one, or would prefer to use your fingers, lie on the bed with your knees up and legs apart or sit up, cross-legged, with your back against the headboard or wall. Try pressing the soles of your feet together to increase tension in the groin.

Some women are so sensitive, they'll stroke themselves through their underwear; some like direct clitoral stimulation, others indirect.

Apply lots of lube to your finger or vulva and use your middle finger to move up and down on the clitoris or do slow circles around the edge if it feels too sensitive. Start by stroking lightly, though you might want to increase the pressure later. Alternatively, you can rub side to side.

Most women prefer a regular rhythm. The clitoris gets dry very easily, so apply more lubricant as you go along or lick your fingers regularly.

RUBBING AGAINST SOMETHING

Remember when you were too young to go "all the way" but used to hump against your partner's leg and hip for stimulation? This is the same technique.

Generally, you hold the object still and move against it. Try lying on your stomach with your genitals pressed firmly into the bed with a pillow or cushion between your legs to rub against. Or lie on your back with a blanket or pillow between your legs and use your hand to hold either side of the pillow to keep the pressure firm. Some women still use their fingers but use a pillow or crunch their legs tightly together to increase the pressure.

You'll need to experiment and maybe "arrange" your genitals so the thrusting feels pleasurable, keeping up a steady rhythm of quite vigorous thrusting until you climax. Placing a cupped hand over the entire genital area and moving it while you're pushing against a pillow is also popular.

When are you going to use it?

Wand vibrators take up a big space in your suitcase when you travel, bullets slip discreetly into your makeup bag. Who's going to be within earshot? Does it need to be super quiet? Do you have nosy kids and grandkids and need it disguised? Wand vibes can easily be passed off as back massagers.

How strong do you want the vibration to be?

Nerve sensitivity alters as you age, so opt for one that's stronger than you need initially and keep it on a low setting. You can always calm it down by putting your hand over it to absorb excessive vibration.

How much do you want to spend?

As a rule of thumb, spend more on products you know you'll use more often—staples like vibrators, lube, etc.—than toys you're buying to add a bit of variety now and then. You don't need to go high budget to get good quality; there are a lot of well-designed, midrange toys made of quality, body-safe materials. Most products are now rechargeable, so you're not forking out for batteries, and they last for years.

Some retailers, including Lovehoney, which makes my line of products, offer a 100-percent money-back guarantee if you're not happy. And yes, this does mean you can take them out of the packaging and try them out properly. (They recycle returned products, just in case you're wondering!) This is handy because it means you get to road-test more expensive products and experiment more.

Where to buy sex toys

If you live in a city, google "female-friendly sex store," and you'll probably find several nonintimidating, pleasant shops staffed by women who actually know what they're talking about and aren't embarrassed talking about sexual needs. Otherwise, as with everything these days, for the best selection, price, and privacy, go online to one of the big retailers.

Other factors to consider
when you're older

- Is it made of nontoxic, body-safe material?

- Is it soft and squeezy to touch, rather than hard?

- Are the buttons easy to press?

- Is it lightweight?

- Is it ergonomic, and does it feel comfortable to hold?

- Is it simple to use? If it's rechargeable, you may need a computer and to be tech-savvy enough to use a USB charger. (It's easy, you just plug it into a slot on your computer.)

- Are the controls easy to see without glasses on?

- How long will it last before it runs out? You don't want it conking out at the crucial moment.

Buy safe

Joan Price is a respected US sex educator who has been writing and blogging about "senior" sex since 2005. (She's written several great books about sex for grown-ups: *Naked at Our Age* is a good one to start with.) Joan is a huge fan of sex toys—but only those that are safe, because "you don't want a product that leaches toxic chemicals anywhere near the delicate tissues of your genitals." Quite. This is what she recommends all women do before buying a sex toy.

- Smell it. If it smells obviously like chemicals or plastic, avoid. A good-quality sex toy should have no smell.

- Check that it's made of nonporous material: glass, silicone, steel, or medical-grade plastics.

- Don't think a condom will stop the nasties. Lots of sex educators (me included) said if you put a condom over the sex toy, you'll protect yourself from any toxic materials. Turns out that's not true. Sorry about that!

TOYS THAT WILL TRANSFORM YOUR SEX LIFE

These are my recommendations for toys, but don't forget about stuff you already have: scarves and stockings are great for blindfolds or tie-ups (make sure you have some strong, sharp scissors in the house, in case you can't undo the knots), well-cut lingerie boosts low body image and spices up any sex session, massage oils and candles set the mood and the scene.

In most cases, I'm going to talk about categories of toys rather than name specific brands.

PRODUCTS YOU NEED

GOOD-QUALITY LUBRICANT

Lube makes just about anything feel better, but it's an absolute must for any type of penetrative sex (fingers, toys, or a penis) post-50. Lubes cling to the vaginal lining the way vaginal secretions do and work to reduce the unwelcome friction that's caused by thin, dry genital tissue.

Water-based lubricants won't eat condoms or your toys, but silicone-based lubricants last longer. Silicone lubes are great if you're sensitive, and they have no flavor. They also dry to a powder finish rather than sticky. Oil-based lubricants are quite moisturizing and also long-lasting but can be a bugger to wash off (you and clothes).

Cheap usually means ghastly when it comes to lubes— they're likely to include highly irritating ingredients like glycerin, petroleum, parabens, nonoxynol-9, propylene glycol, benzocaine, and chlorhexidine gluconate. Also avoid mineral-based oil lubes, which aren't body friendly. Spend more and read the labels. Carefully.

KEGEL BALLS OR A KEGEL EXERCISER SYSTEM

Apart from having regular intercourse or investing in some type of vaginal rejuvenation using lasers (see page 68 for more on this), regular Kegel exercises are still one of the most effective ways to keep your sex organs fit and healthy. An added bonus: the more toned and tight your pelvic floor muscles, the more intense orgasms feel.

If you've had children, you'll have been lectured on the importance of doing regular pelvic-floor exercises. They basically involve repetitively squeezing and releasing the same muscles you'd squeeze to stop the flow of urine.

They're more effective if you have something to squeeze around because it forces you to do the exercise properly (squeezing the PC muscle rather than the muscles in you anus and thighs).

Kegel toner balls, which you insert high into the vagina, are weighted to help improve muscle tone even further during your genital workout. You can buy them as one single ball, doubles, or sets that increase in size and weight. Some vibrate, to turn you on during the "workout," or you can go high-tech with toners that use electrical pulses or track your progress on your smartphone.

TOYS YOU'LL WANT

WARMING GEL

Warming gels contain products like arginine and menthol, which work to enhance sensation and maximize climax potential during solo play or sex with your partner. You rub it around the clitoris. Gels create a warming sensation and increase blood flow to the area.

WAND VIBRATORS

This type of vibrator is top of the list for good reason. Wand vibes are powerful—and lots of us need stronger vibration than we used to. They cover a bigger area than other targeted vibes—good news when your nerve endings aren't as sensitive as they were—and they're great for external stimulation, if delicate tissue or dryness is a problem.

They can be battery-operated, rechargeable, or powered by electricity. Wands you plug into the wall are a one-time investment (I've had mine for 15 years). The vibration is steady, consistent, and teeth-chatteringly strong—hell, you really can use it to massage your shoulders! Electric vibrators were invented before irons and vacuum cleaners—good to see someone had their priorities right!—and the Original Magic Wand is still the most popular vibrator in the world.

Corded electric wands tend to be heavier to hold than rechargeable or battery vibes and are more expensive. But panic not. There are plenty of well-designed, noncorded wands out there that still pack a punch.

BULLET VIBES

They look like large tampons, are tiny enough to take anywhere, but are powerful enough to deliver good, strong clitoral stimulation. They're also perfect for caressing nipples, around the rim of your bottom—anywhere you'd like a bit of a buzz really.

Inexpensive, versatile, and completely nonthreatening in shape (nothing phallic here), bullets are a perfect choice if you've never used a sex toy before. You can also use it to get yourself in the mood before sex. If you want a head start, head to the bathroom with one in your pocket and let it work its magic.

CLITORAL VIBRATORS

Anything that vibrates is essentially a clitoral vibrator, but there are targeted vibes, specifically designed for this purpose. Bullets are clitoral vibes. As are pebble vibes that sit in the palm of your hand. They're small, oval-shaped, and curved to cover the labial area. If you find your clitoris has gotten more sensitive over time, they'll suit you because the vibration is gentler.

Clitoral suction vibrators stimulate the clitoris—without even touching it. They use new air technology that produces gentle sucking and soft vibrations, providing an entirely different stimulation than normal vibrators. The most famous is the Womanizer, though other brands are starting to emerge. It's another style that's great to try if you're supersensitive. But stick to the lowest settings.

RABBIT VIBRATORS

A rabbit is what springs to mind when most people picture a vibrator. If you're over 50 and not interested in using a sex toy, this is probably why. When you're young and superkeen on penetration, a large penis-shaped shaft that whirls around to stimulate your vaginal wall looks like heaven. When you're older, all those fancy beads twirling around just look painful. The vibrating "ears" of the rabbit are positioned to work on the clitoris while the shaft is inserted. In my opinion, there are other vibrators that are better suited for older women (see above), but if this all sounds appealing, go for it!

THE BEST TOYS FOR HIM

Decreased blood flow makes it harder for men to get and sustain an erection when they're older. Like us, he also takes longer to get aroused and needs extra stimulation. Happily, sex toys check lots of those "can help" boxes.

A MASTURBATORY SLEEVE OR "STROKER"

This is a simple but ingenious invention that has revolutionized masturbation and foreplay. They've been around forever (you may have heard of the brand Fleshlight, which are strokers that

look like fake vaginas). Today's strokers ar
tubes, usually textured—that mold to th
penis.

You simply put a dab of lube inside, s
and use one hand to slide it up and dow
amateur hand job into something quite spectacu

PENIS RINGS

These come in many different forms, but all slip over the penis
to sit snugly at the base. The idea is that they hold the blood
in the chambers to keep him harder—with varying success.
Lots of men like using them, though. They feel like someone's
squeezing him, always nice, and can help delay orgasm and
make it feel more powerful.

PROSTATE MASSAGERS

The prostate gland might be a source of worry for lots of older
men but it's also a sexual hot spot, otherwise known as the
male G-spot.

Prostate massagers—which come in myriad shapes and
designs, vibrating and nonvibrating—are proving to be a big hit
with older men. They not only help him achieve fierce orgasms,
but they also help to stimulate blood flow to the penis, which
can mean firmer erections.

Read the guide on how to give him a prostate massage
(page 149) before using a prostate massager for the first time.
You'll find tips on how to prepare it for insertion and the area
you're aiming for.

Once inserted, you (or he) simply hold the end of the massager
and start by rubbing it around the area inside, discovering

it feels best. Generally, the more pressure you apply to prostate gland, the more aroused he'll feel. Also try an up-and-down motion, done rapidly or slowly, and add oral or hand stimulation for an orgasm he won't forget in a hurry.

TOYS TO USE TOGETHER

A SLIMLINE CLASSIC VIBE

Think old-school: vibrators that are slim and cylindrical with a rounded top. They're cheap, the shape carries vibration well, so they're strong, and best of all, they're couple friendly. He'll like it because they're small but look enough like a penis for him to convince himself this must be your idea of the "perfect" penis size.

They're easy and nonintrusive to hold between you, on your clitoris, if you do want to have intercourse. You can use it on all your hot spots—nipples, bottom, wherever—and because they're small, they're good for gentle penetration.

BUTT PLUGS

Not only can butt plugs help him achieve an erection, but if vaginal penetration makes you sore, your bottom provides an alternative means of stimulation. Anal stimulation is something lots of people have a negative knee-jerk reaction to, but once tried, it often makes it onto the "regular activity" list.

Butt plugs are a nonthreatening place to start. They're shaped like little penises who've eaten too much—bigger in the middle with a flared end (to stop it disappearing up you-know-where;

the vagina has an "end" that the rectum effectively doesn't). After you insert it (using lots of lube and waiting until the person is highly aroused), you simply leave it there during oral sex or intercourse to add an erotic edge. They make you feel pleasantly "filled up" and provide pressure on everything else (the rectum shares a wall with the vagina). You can buy vibrating butt plugs or insert a slim vibrator a little way to see if you like the sensation (without letting go, unless it has a flared end).

DILDOS AND PEGGING KITS

They're designed for vaginal and anal penetration (if they have a flared base) and are superversatile. You can buy dildos in all sorts of materials and, best, in all sorts of sizes. (The difference between a dildo and a vibrator, by the way, is that dildos don't vibrate.)

If he's having erection problems and you're a fan of penetration, they take the pressure off because you have a "penis" at the ready. If you like penetration but his penis now feels too big, buy one in a smaller size. Strap-on dildos (sometimes called "pegging kits") are also an option. The harness attaches around your hips and thighs, and the dildo sits inside it. An instant erection for him, or you wear it to "peg" him. (Pegging is when a woman anally penetrates a man wearing a strap-on dildo.)

Dildos are perfect for role-playing. The prettiest come in glass and you can heat them up or cool them down to roll over the whole body.

SOFT BONDAGE KITS

When libidos are sluggish, it takes more than missionary to kick-start them again. Tie-up games can revive routine sex lives, shifting power and adding a welcome frisson of excitement. Pink, fluffy handcuffs can feel silly on older wrists, and steel is cold and unforgiving. "Soft" bondage kits are made from comfortable material and usually attach with Velcro so they're easy to put on and take off. They're inexpensive, too.

VIBRATING LOVE EGGS

Choose one that's small, made of silicone, and with a remote, and you've got yourself an impressive tease toy. Use lube, insert the egg high into the vagina, then hand the controls over to your lover so they can turn it and you on—whenever and wherever they choose.

Lots of women who have issues with penetration can use love eggs. Unlike a penis that thrusts back and forth, the egg just sits in place, buzzing away gently. (If it feels uncomfortable, it might be because it's not inserted high enough.)

G-SPOT VIBES

If you've got issues with painful sex and penetration is difficult, steer clear. Otherwise, give these a go for a totally different, highly intense orgasm.

G-spot vibrators are hugely popular for one very good reason: it's notoriously difficult to reach the infamous hot spot using fingers or a penis. These vibes are curved and sculpted specifically for this purpose and great to use for both sexes. (There's still contention over whether or not there is a "G-spot," but the front wall of the vagina [under your belly] is definitely acutely responsive to stimulation. When I say the "G-spot," I mean this area.)

You use a G-spot vibe differently than others. Lie on your back with knees pulled up and a pillow under your buttocks, lie on your tummy, or get on hands and knees. Use lots of lube, then gently insert the vibrator about 1 to 3 inches inside. Aim it at the roof of the vagina (like you're aiming for your stomach) and move the vibe back and forth or in circles, keeping the pressure firm and repetitive.

Don't panic if you feel like you want to pee: you won't. It's because you're pressing on the urethra (the tube that carries urine). Relax into the sensation until it passes and you'll (hopefully!) climax.

WEDGES, RAMPS, AND OTHER SEX FURNITURE

Your genitals are in great shape, it's the rest of you that's going to pot? If you've got bad knees or back issues, stiff joints or arthritis, do a search for "sex furniture" (or check out Liberator, the most famous brand). Sex furniture includes everything from luxurious (expensive) chaise longues to odd-shaped cushions that provide support where it's needed. "Wedges" and "ramps"—imagine a slice of cake—slip under bottoms, knees, or elbows to help get you into position for sex or to help make it more comfortable.

If you don't want to invest, take inspiration and find sex props you already have in your house. Simply putting firm pillows under various parts of each of you can mean the difference between a nervous, anxious sex session—worried your back's going to go or your knees give out—and one that's comfortable and enjoyable.

DEBUNKING MYTHS ABOUT SEX TOYS

As a regular user of sex toys for the last 42 years (yikes!), I can happily reassure you on all of the following.

Will vibrators make you numb? No, and they won't make you less sensitive, either. Quite the opposite, actually: vibrators keep the blood flowing to the genitals, keeping them healthy. They're quick, too: lots of us can go from zero to a climax within three to five minutes using a vibrator.

Are sex toys as good as the real thing? If the "real thing" is a man's penis, I think you'll find a lot of sex toys are better. Intercourse is one of the most unreliable ways for women to orgasm. Only 20 to 30 percent of women orgasm with a partner through penetrative sex, but most women orgasm every single time when they masturbate with a vibrator. "I had my first orgasm at 57 using a vibrator," says Erica, now 63. "I cried. I didn't even know females could orgasm until I was quite old. Now I don't mind if there's a gap between relationships. I have my massager."

Will you end up preferring your vibrator to having sex with your partner? Quite frankly, you might when you first use one. But vibrators can't make you laugh, watch TV with you, or give you a cuddle, so it's unlikely you'll be showing him the door and snuggling up with your wand vibe. On the other hand, if you're staying in a rubbish relationship purely for the sex, a vibrator might well convince you you're better off single. This is a good thing.

Are sex toys unnatural? Really? I suspect you do lots of things that are "unnatural." Like use electricity. Drive a car. Put your food in a fridge. Vibrators are one of the world's greatest inventions. Be thankful, not suspicious!

9

HOW TO SURVIVE

IN A

SEXLESS RELATIONSHIP

SEX STOPS IN RELATIONSHIPS FOR all sorts of reasons. Sometimes it's a natural decline in your libido that makes you both not want sex anymore—and you're both perfectly happy to wave it farewell. Other times, one hangs up their skates and the other is still very much wanting to whiz around the ice rink.

Mismatched libidos—when one of you wants sex much more than the other—play hell with the best relationships. But if you want to see true chaos, try telling a partner who thoroughly enjoys sex that it will never be available again. Yet plenty of people do.

Our culture has never been more tolerant of sex, more permissive or accepting of just about every permutation, yet we're in the middle of a worldwide sex recession. And none of us are immune. The number of adult Americans who reported no sexual activity in the last year reached an all-time high in 2018. According to a report from the University of Chicago General Social Survey, 23 percent of adults—nearly a quarter of Americans surveyed— had not had sex in the past year, up significantly from 2008, when the percentage of American adults not having sex was at around 9 percent. And it's primarily young men between the ages of 18 and 30 that are driving this trend: 28 percent of young men reported not having had sex in the past year, as opposed to 18 percent of young women. The sex recession appears to be global, with Australia, Finland, and the Netherlands all seeing similar declines. In Japan, in 2015, 43 percent of people aged 18 to 34 were virgins.

There are myriad reasons why the world is going off sex. Every couple is unique, but there are certain things that affect all of us.

THE REASONS WHY YOU'VE STOPPED HAVING SEX

Technology. One of the biggest culprits today is technology. Twenty years ago, most couples used to have sex at 10:24 p.m. on a Saturday night. Now, we're lying on the sofa, binging on Netflix. When we finally do get to bed, instead of turning to each other, we flick through social media or the news to find out what's going on in the world. Lots, it turns out. Which means not a lot going on in the bedroom.

Too busy. Personally, I think "no time" is an excuse way more often than it's a real reason. We all manage to find time for TV and social media. But there are genuine cases where one or both of you are emotionally and physically exhausted by the demands of life.

The porn bubble. Solo sex requires little effort and zero upkeep, couple sex requires quite a bit of both. It's easy to get into the habit of masturbating for five minutes while watching porn twice a week and that's both of you done.

Porn will always be popular because humans are lazy—couples will embrace "sexbots" for the same reason. We'll be able to fine-tune our sex robots to cater to our every need with little input required from us. A lot less hassle than pesky, demanding fellow humans.

A lifetime of bad sex. Some people aren't good at telling partners what works for them, so they put up with years of ineffectual technique. Others are bullied into having sex with partners they don't even like, let alone love. If sex is not a pleasant experience and makes you feel bad about yourself, why wouldn't you want it to stop?

Bored with sex. You've done it thousands of times already and simply lost interest. Netflix changes its content constantly, which is more than you can say about the average couple's sex routine.

Sexual dysfunctions and health issues. Erection problems, painful sex, general ill health, and flexibility issues—most of these things are treatable, but many people don't seek help.

Low self-esteem. If you have no confidence—don't like how you look and don't feel remotely desirable—you're unlikely to think of sex as a fun thing to do.

Depression or anxiety. More than 35 million Americans, four million people in the UK, and three million Australians are long-term users of antidepressants. What's a common side effect of taking these drugs? Low libido.

Loss of desire. Even if you love each other, even if you used to have really good sex, desire for sex does fall the older we get. If you seriously don't think it's going to happen to you, it can come as quite a shock when it does.

Relationship problems. I find it astonishing when couples believe their love and sex life aren't connected. "I don't know why we're not having sex anymore," one woman told me. Two breaths later, she complained that she and her husband seemed perpetually angry at each other. "Not having sex is making it worse," she said.

It's a classic lose-lose scenario: feeling angry stops you from having sex; not having sex makes you feel even angrier. You can't expect good sex if your relationship has been shitty for years. Infidelity is another efficient way to cut the best sex life off at the knees.

No one to have sex with. Judging by many responses to a questionnaire I asked single women to fill in, there's a distinct lack of ready, willing, and able men to have sex with once you head into the second half of your life. (Plenty on this in chapter 11.)

It probably *won't* be because of lesbian bed death if you're a woman who likes sex with women. There's little evidence to support the concept that if you put two women together, sex dies off quicker than if a woman is paired with a man. In fact, a recent study found lesbians have more orgasms than straight or bisexual women and more satisfying sex. If anything, two women over 50 are more likely to come up with inventive scenarios to keep sex going than agree for it to stop, because they aren't as penetration focused.

WON'T IT JUST SORT ITSELF OUT WITH TIME?

Do you also believe in unicorns? If you've stopped having sex, it's highly unlikely you're going to spontaneously turn to each other after several sexless years and suddenly exclaim, "Can you believe it? We forgot to have sex for five years! Let's do it now!"

A US survey of 1,000 people found that while a small portion of married people who've experienced a "dead bedroom" get back on track, lots don't. Thirty-nine percent said dry spells lasted between one and five years.

What usually happens when one person seems disinterested is, the other makes a bit of an effort to get things started again but stops trying if their efforts aren't enthusiastically welcomed. Advances are rarely welcome if there's a problem you're putting your head in the sand about. The initiator then gives up and finds something else to amuse themselves with—the gym, a new hobby, a new job, grandkids. It's alarmingly easy to forget how good sex can be when you're not having it, and how quickly you both adjust to the new norm. Sex disappears further and further into the distance and you hardly notice it's gone. It's daunting having sex when you haven't done it in months. Terrifying if you haven't done it in years.

Most sexless marriages also remain sexless because of the Westermarck effect (named after a Finnish anthropologist). Westermarck believed humans have an innate tendency to lose desire for people they live with for a sustained period of time if they aren't having sex with them. Living together as friends means you begin to feel like siblings. Sex feels "wrong" and intensely awkward, so you avoid it.

It doesn't really matter what your reason for stopping initially was. Once you have stopped having sex for longer than a year, it nearly always stays that way unless one or both of you tackle the problem head-on.

WHAT DOES IT FEEL LIKE TO HAVE SEX RARELY OR NOT AT ALL?

"I would never tell my friends we don't have sex anymore. People assume things. Is he gay? Is he secretly having an affair? Are you about to get a divorce? What about you're just not that bothered about sex anymore?"

"I'd rather have a partner who doesn't have sex than one who can't keep it in his pants and is unfaithful or watches porn for hours at a time."

"I'm 60. I've had enough sex to last me a lifetime. It's never been my favorite part of a relationship. My husband has had 40 years of me having sex to keep him happy, now it's my turn. I really don't care if he gets it elsewhere. I don't want to know and I want him to be discreet, but if that stops him hassling me, great."

"Once he started having erection problems, sex became less and less interesting to my husband. He hated what was happening and Viagra didn't agree with him. He's never been a hugely sexual person, and I suspect his testosterone is low because he's not a competitive, driven man. We talk about having sex, but he's always got a reason why we shouldn't do it. The reasons are lame and it's really because it's too much hassle. Too many hurdles to jump. It's fine but I do feel he's forgotten about me, that I might want sex for the intimacy. I've always had most of my orgasms through oral sex, so there's no reason why I can't still enjoy it."

"We used to have great sex at the start. We'd go to bed for hours at a time. Take a bottle of wine and make love for hours. Twenty years on, we'd rather do something else like watch a movie or go out to lunch. We still have sex but it's rare and doesn't last very long. Sex is like everything else in life. There's a time when it's important in your life and there's a time when it's not. We're both perfectly happy with where we are now. Maybe later, we'll rediscover it again."

FIND YOUR NORMAL

When does a marriage become "sexless"? What if you still do it but only once a month or once a year? Officially, it used to be your marriage was considered sexless if you had sex less than 10 times a year. This definition was way too narrow and it's now been changed to "a marriage with little or no sexual activity."

Some people feel sex-starved if they have sex once a week. Others will have an enjoyable sex session twice a year and still rate their sex life as highly satisfying. I know plenty of long-term couples over 50 who have sex every two months and would bristle with indignation if I branded their relationship "sexless." The right amount of sex for both of you has nothing to do with how often you're having it and everything to do with what makes you both happy. I can't stress this enough.

Yes, sex is good for you—massively beneficial—in lots of ways. I have gone over a myriad of emotional and physical reasons why over the course of this book. But lots of couples thrive in no-sex or low-sex relationships. Sex isn't the only thing that's important in life. "It's not how often you have it, it's knowing you could have it. And knowing your partner would want it as well," one happily married man in his sixties told me. They have sex once a month and it works for them. There is no "normal." Once a week appears to be the magic number to reap the benefits sex brings, but that's a figure for all couples. It doesn't take into account age and stage. How long you've been together, what else is happening in your lives, what sex means to each of you, and a dozen other variables need to be factored in. Love, playfulness, affection—these things also bring intimacy to relationships and are equally as important as sex.

For those who relate to numbers, a US study of more than 70,000 people (*The Normal Bar*'s online survey) included 8,240 participants who were 50 or over. Thirty-three percent of those couples said they rarely or never had sex. One quarter of those rated themselves as being "extremely happy."

There is most definitely a strong correlation between sexual intimacy and sense of well-being. A recent study by the International Society for Sexual Medicine of 3,000 men and 4,000 women, most in their mid-sixties, found those who had sex in the past year reported enjoying their lives more. But if you're having a wonderful life with your partner, you're great friends, demonstrative, have a laugh, share the same interests, enjoy time with your kids, friends, and family, and lead a full, interesting life, sex is the icing on the cake and not the main ingredient. With one enormous caveat: so long as both of you agree.

One thing you must also always remember: decent, regular sex goes a long way to smooth over the not-so-perfect parts of our relationships. If you do decide to stop doing it, you need to be extra vigilant with relationship "housekeeping."

WHAT COULD MEN DO TO MAKE WOMEN WANT SEX MORE?

"Spend more time being affectionate and attentive. I really love a good, relaxing massage and it will often lead to sex. I need to feel emotionally connected to want sex."

"Middle-aged women often say they feel invisible and are no longer seen as sexually attractive. Anything that lets us know we still are is important. I have several friends whose marriages have ended after the guy left them for a much younger woman. Women feel vulnerable."

"Listen more. As a woman gets older, there are so many narratives in their heads. Menopause is a big factor. So is dealing with getting older."

"Give more compliments. We're not getting as many as we used to. Any kind of positive reinforcement about our looks, our feelings, how attractive we are, really helps."

"More romance. We need lots of stroking and teasing: stop going straight for my clitoris."

WHAT COULD WOMEN DO TO MAKE MEN WANT SEX MORE?

"Reassure him it's not all about performance. It's about connecting on all sorts of levels and not just via intercourse."

"Give them compliments. He's not as confident as he was."

"Pay attention to their needs. Men, too, need to feel wanted. I think men need more emotional connection as they get older and get better at relationships."

"I've never met a man who didn't want sex. I've never met a man who wasn't happy in bed with whatever he got."

"Men also struggle with the reality of the physical change that comes with middle age and the waning of their sexual prowess."

WHAT TO DO WHEN . . . YOU BOTH DON'T WANT TO HAVE SEX ANYMORE

Couples who happily draw the line under sex have often never really been that sexual. Throw in some of the issues that typically affect people over 50 and that can be enough to extinguish what flame there was.

Some of us power energetically through the years, others slow down and start to feel worn out. Different things become important. When you're young, swapping sex for a country walk or gardening sounds bonkers. As you sidestep, nervously, toward 60, you start to get it. What excites you post-50 isn't necessarily what excited you in the first half of your life.

Whatever the reason for you both deciding to become sexless, there is one factor that will dictate how your relationship will be from now on. You must—and I mean must—acknowledge what it is you're doing. If you don't, your relationship is vulnerable.

Some couples who want to stop having sex withdraw everything. There's no kissing, no flirting or touching, no sexy lingerie or even sexy outfits. They avert their eyes when couples have sex on television and avoid any conversation that involves sex. You don't want to have sex, so you avoid anything and everything that might lead to it. Not only does this kill any desire you might have been able to resurrect, but it also ruins your relationship. Take away touch and affection, and you are effectively separating while living together.

Some couples do this when they really would like to split but neither wants to compromise their lifestyle by divorcing or they can't bear to hurt the kids. If this is you, do both of you a favor and get it out into the open. Acknowledge that this is what you're doing and you're both happy doing it, and you can get on with your lives, without sneaking around. Who knows? You might end up great friends. Pretending all is normal when it's not is just exhausting—and pointless—for everyone. Your kids know what's going on, they aren't stupid.

But even if you don't fall into that category—you love each other desperately and can't imagine anything worse than living without each other—you still have to have "the talk." Some extremely close couples say the conversation doesn't have to be traumatic or even that long. "We looked at each other in bed one night and I said, 'Do you mind that we don't have sex anymore?' He replied, 'Not at all. So long as we cuddle, that's fine with me.' And that was that."

But there does need to be a moment when you both completely understand, without a shadow of doubt, that you are both now going to have a relationship that doesn't include sex. Once you've done that, keep the love side extra happy by doing all of the following:

Double the affection. Once you both know that a touch isn't a prelude to wanting sex, you can relax. Hold hands, cuddle, give each other kisses, and do it often.

Keep being playful. Not having sex doesn't mean you can't sleep naked, cuddled up. Have fun. Your sexual hot spots aren't contaminated just because you don't want to take it further. Slap him on the bottom. Love that he gives your bottom a squeeze or admires your cleavage. Give his penis a friendly yank now and then.

Keep the discussion going. Check in to make sure you're both still happy with the situation. You might just find, having taken the pressure off, the idea of sex becomes quite appealing again. Be aware, one of you might change their mind. If this does happen and your partner announces they do want sex after all, don't panic.

Separate beds can work. It's not a sexy concept, but there are many reasons why couples sleep apart. A recent study found up to 200,000 Australian couples now sleep in separate beds because of their partner's snoring, restlessness, and blanket stealing. The "sleep divorce" has strengthened relationships rather than harmed them.

YOUR PARTNER DOESN'T WANT TO HAVE SEX ANYMORE AND YOU DO

The crucial question here is why—the reason dictates what you should do about it. If your partner no longer wants to have sex because of something that's obvious and not their fault—they've got a life-changing illness, or are struggling with health issues, going through a rough time, or depressed or stressed over a life event that's out of their control—this is a completely different scenario than them simply deciding "Right, that's me. I'm done." But, even then, there's usually some wiggle room.

Sex as you used to have it might be impossible, but some type of sex might well be achievable. Where there's a will, there's a way. I used to do workshops with people who suffer from brittle bone disease. Some were severely disabled, wheelchair-bound, and with bones so delicate they would break from a sneeze. The average person says no to sex when they have a cold or a "fat day." Some of the people I met were in considerable pain pretty much all of the time: going to the bathroom required major effort. Yet, here they were, at a workshop that would help them find a way to make sexual connections, despite their disability. It was a humbling exercise and a profound lesson in how important being sexual is to human beings. It also makes our excuses for not having sex seem rather pathetic.

If your partner's no longer physically fit enough to have intercourse, they may still be well enough to satisfy you. Can they use their hands or tongue to pleasure you? Can they hold a sex toy to stimulate you? At the very least, they can be in the room when you masturbate, making them part of it all, telling you how hot you look when you do it. (Mental illness is quite another story and a situation only you know and can make decisions about.) Just because they don't want anything sexual being done to them, are they open to still sexually stimulating you?

Other good questions to ask yourself when your partner seems to no longer want sex: Are they at least willing to explore options? Do they want to make you happy and do what they can to meet your needs? Are they willing to talk about the problem and try to fix it? If the answer to all of these questions is yes, it might simply be a case of thinking outside the box and coming up with imaginative solutions.

Two likely scenarios

Sometimes sex stops for no big reason. You just started having it less (you're busy with the kids, working hard, juggling elderly parents, etc.), and it trickled down from once a week to once a month to once to never. You've tried initiating but your partner always seems to have an excuse, and you don't want to rock the boat by making it real and saying, "How come you don't want to have sex anymore?" If your relationship is fine and it's just your sex life that's dead, you've probably been looking after yourself by masturbating and hoping like hell that, one day, things will get back on track. If you're still joking about not "doing it," it doesn't feel like a big problem.

You're right—it's certainly not as big a problem as the other likely scenario. It's when sex stops and your partner withdraws and refuses to talk about it at all that problems really start. Your first thought might be that they don't find you attractive anymore. Feeling undesirable isn't the best feeling in the world. Following close on the heels of that is that they're having an affair or want out of the relationship. Toss feeling unloved and unwanted on top of undesirable. "Is he gay?" might get tossed into the bubbling pot of paranoia as well. (Or "Is she straight?" if you're lesbian.) Listen, it might be one of those reasons. But if you're with a man and he's over 50, and he used to love sex but now avoids it and refuses to talk about it, it nearly always means he's having erection problems and is too embarrassed to admit it.

What happens when men stop having sex

A lot of men with ED (erectile dysfunction) would rather not have sex ever again than fess up to such a shameful secret. And I'm talking otherwise open, communicative men who are happy talking about virtually anything else. There's a whole chapter on this to help you talk through this issue and find solutions, so if you think ED might well be the reason, off you go to page 131.

Loss of desire, simply not feeling like sex anymore, can also be devastating because the conventional script says a man should always be up for sex, regardless of age. The reality is: "In my office these days, it's far more common for a wife to bring her husband in because he has gone missing in bed than the other way around," says sex therapist Stephen Snyder. Not wanting sex is emasculating.

Whether it's him saying no or you, a lack of sex often impacts men more. Sex doesn't just give men orgasms, it provides intimacy. Women are better at seeking affection and closeness when they need it. They'll ask for a hug—lots of men won't, even when they're upset, for fear of looking "weak." They initiate sex instead: it's their way of saying "I need to feel close to you." Men need connection and emotional closeness just as much as we do, and if sex was his main source of this, stopping it leaves him feeling lonely and isolated.

What now?

Most of you will be in one of the two scenarios I described earlier. Either sex has stopped and you don't know what to do to restart it again, and your partner doesn't seem interested when you initiate, but your relationship seems fine otherwise. Or you have no clue why sex has stopped, your partner won't talk to you about it and is no longer loving. This is when, as well as feeling unlovable, unattractive, and rejected, you feel bewildered, confused, and frustrated.

If things are so bad the entire relationship is on its knees, then rescuing the physical part really is the least of your worries. This is a crisis. See a therapist or counselor as soon as possible, and if your partner won't come with you, go solo. Either that or call it quits.

The solution for the rest of you is the same. Like it or not (and most of you won't), you have to talk.

HOW TO TACKLE THE ELEPHANT IN THE ROOM

No, there really isn't another way. Yes, you can do it. So read this, take a few deep breaths, and get on with having that honest conversation. Here's how to prepare.

Before the talk

Don't feel guilty for wanting sex. If you're in a monogamous relationship, there is an obligation on each of you to keep each other happy sexually. It's part of the deal. If sex is important to you, great!

Don't bury your own desire just because your partner has. Women are great at seeing their partner's perspective and bending to other people's needs, but their needs are just as important as their partners'.

Has your partner noticed how long it's been? If your partner genuinely is too busy or stressed to register that sex has gone AWOL, simply pointing out how long it's been and how much you miss it may be all that's required.

If sex has become awkward—which it quickly does when you don't do it on a regular basis—neither of you are going to want to rush back for a repeat. If your partner's not great at expressing their feelings, they might be desperate to resume having sex, but unsure of how to talk to you about it to clear the air. Once you start, the rest might be easy.

What type of sex do you want? This seems like an odd question, but it isn't. Yes, I know you want to have sex again. But how often? What sort of sex? What do you miss the most? Is it the cuddles and pillow talk, the intimacy of lying there together naked? Or is it the orgasms? Maybe both. Do you want sex to include intercourse? Or are you happy with foreplay? Do you want to try new things? Use sex toys?

Think about what your ideal sex session would involve. Do you want to talk first? Do something romantic like go out to dinner or have a bath together? How would sex start? How would it end?

Once you've come up with a detailed scenario, think about what your partner used to like. Try to include things you know did it for them in the past so it's appealing to both of you. You don't have to launch into this much detail during the initial talk, but if they ask questions, it's good to have thought it through, and it will be super helpful later.

Decide on a good time to talk. If they've been avoiding talking about sex, no time will be a good time. Their reaction to you finally daring to tackle the issue might well be to become angry, storm out, pick a fight, cry, or clam up and refuse to speak. Expect any or all of these reactions. Sometimes, the first talk doesn't go so well, but often, they'll go away and think through what you said and be ready to talk again in a day or so.

Even so, increase the odds of it going well by choosing a time when you're both relaxed and in a place you know your partner feels comfortable. Don't do it in the bedroom. Definitely don't do it when you've just initiated sex and been turned down. You both need to be calm.

Having the talk

Flattery will get you everywhere. Pitch it so you're saying how attractive you find them, how much you miss the great sex you used to have, and you'll get a much better reaction—so say all the men I interviewed about this. Men are suckers for compliments: lay them on thick and he'll be far more open to listening to what else you have to say.

Start with something simple. Say, "Look, I wanted to talk to you about something. I love you and love our relationship and miss having sex. Have you noticed we're not having it anymore? How do you feel about that?" Or, if things really aren't good, "I'm worried about our relationship. I don't feel like we're as close. We don't talk as much and we're not having sex anymore. Can we have a talk about why?"

Don't panic if they get angry. Anger is just fear. They're also embarrassed. The aim is to get them talking; shouting is better than silence, and defensiveness is better than indifference.

Count to 10 and try not to react if they say something like, "Well, if you didn't spend so much, maybe I wouldn't have to work so hard." Or they become really nasty and resort to personal insults like, "If you lost some weight, I might be interested."

Talking about sex problems is one of the most stressful conversations for most couples, particularly men. Your partner will be feeling under attack and the first instinct is to fight back. If they immediately apologize and look mortified for having been rude, forgive and move forward. But don't let them blame it all on you. If they're being inexcusably horrible, tell them you'll talk to them later when they calm down.

Keep it simple. If your partner is mortified by the conversation and clearly struggling just to be in the room with you, it's pointless trying to turn it into a long discussion. At least it's out there and can no longer be ignored. Give them an option. Say, "Are you happy to talk about it now? Or would you like to think about it and then we talk later?"

Remember to listen. You've had time to prepare for this and have lots to say. But don't be surprised if, once you've started talking, your partner does, too. Just because they haven't brought it up themselves doesn't mean they haven't been thinking about it as well.

Listen to what they have to say. Really listen. Repeat back to them what it is you've heard to make sure you've got it right.

Use "I," not "you." Say, "I think sex is important," "I need sex to feel close to you." Don't say, "You might be done with sex, but I'm not. Where does that leave me?" It sounds accusatory and blaming.

Talk feelings first, then solutions. Don't skip over the feelings to get to the fix-it part too quickly. This is an emotional moment. You'll both be feeling vulnerable and it's important that you both feel heard.

After the talk

Some partners are relieved and happy when they're forced into discussing something they've been avoiding. The talk ends up going on for a long time, wine gets opened, you reminisce about the sex you used to have, and you come up with some great ideas about how to reintroduce it.

Other times, it clears the air but also becomes crystal clear that your partner has no interest at all in having sex again on a regular basis or at all. If that's the case, you both need time to think about the next steps before talking through the possible options (see page 92).

If you decide you're fine with that, make it clear you're willing to skip sex but not affection and cuddles. They may be scared to touch you in case you'll think they want more: tackle it now, so it doesn't become an issue. You'll also benefit from reading the tips on page 189 about how to keep a sexless relationship happy.

Some partners simply refuse to talk at all. They'll walk out of the room whenever you bring it up and close down completely. Or the talk feels so hopeless or so one-sided in effort, it nails the coffin shut on what you now realize was an already dead relationship. Therapy could be useful if this is what's happened. If your partner won't go with you, it's still worth going yourself. Or it might be time to walk away.

Therapy is also useful even if you're both quite optimistic you can solve it together. It's not easy resuming sex after a long time without it. Try my suggestions, but if you do feel like you're struggling, a few good sessions with a great sex therapist will be money well spent.

YOUR OPTIONS WHEN YOUR PARTNER NO LONGER WANTS TO HAVE SEX WITH YOU

Have solo sex, watch porn, fantasize, use sex toys

In other words, satisfy yourself by stimulating yourself without other people being involved. This works for lots of people—more so when the partner who doesn't want sex makes it clear they're happy for all of this to happen. Not so successful when the person denying you sex also disapproves of you masturbating. Really?

Have nonreciprocal sex

They can still sexually stimulate you by giving hand jobs or oral sex or using sex toys. My husband laughed when I told him I was suggesting this option. "Men won't go for that—they're selfish," he said. "They think, *What's in it for me?*, and there's nothing in it for him if he's doing stuff to her but she's not doing anything back."

"What about giving her pleasure? Making her happy?" I countered.

"Good luck," he said.

Next time around, I'm coming back as a man. Women are so used to giving without receiving anything back, it doesn't sound strange at all to me. If one of you really wants Italian takeout and the other doesn't, sometimes you eat some pasta when you'd rather have a salad. It's all part of the constant compromises you make when you're a couple.

How is this any different? If your partner decides they've had enough sex and don't want anymore, surely the very least they can do is push themselves a little out of their comfort zone? Giving you an orgasm even if they don't want one surely isn't too much to ask?

Have unapproved sex on the side

You might decide you want to stay with your partner but intend to satisfy your sexual urges through one-night stands, sign up for a website that caters to married people seeking sex with others, use sex workers, or have an ongoing affair. I understand why you'd go for this choice. Just don't kid yourself that your partner will forgive you if they find out.

Lots of people think it's perfectly fine to stop having sex even if their partner isn't happy about it. You might think it's obvious you'll seek sex elsewhere, but they may not *agree*. You always risk losing your relationship over infidelity, regardless of the circumstances.

Receive unspoken approval to have sex with others

This often takes the form of your partner saying, "Do what you need to do, but I don't want to know about it," when you finally get them to acknowledge your sex life is nonexistent.

Have approved sex on the side

Sometimes, particularly if one of you isn't well enough to have sex anymore, the other will say it's OK if you have sex with others. This generally happens with couples who loved having sex together and can no longer continue for whatever reason (often health issues). Trouble is, if you still adore your partner, you often don't want to have sex with anyone else.

It's also an option when the relationship morphs into pure friendship but one of you wants to remain sexual. The other wants the companionship, stability, and financial security of a relationship so agrees to put up with you having sex elsewhere in return for you staying in a sexless relationship.

There are nearly always rules with approved sex outside the relationship. It's sensible to agree that it won't be with anyone you both know. Sometimes, couples insist that it can't be with the same person more than once. Nearly all hope that it will be a purely sexual relationship with no feelings involved, but few are silly enough to send their partner out the door into the arms of another warm body without accepting that they are putting the primary relationship in peril.

Leave the relationship

If you're a person who enjoys sex and loves the intimacy and connection and all the other profoundly extraordinary things that sex provides, no sex is usually a deal-breaker. In that case, it's kinder on both of you to separate and let each other find someone more compatible, rather than try to flail along unhappy and resentful.

HOW TO RECONNECT SEXUALLY AFTER A DROUGHT

The two programs I am going to suggest here are frequently recommended by the world's top sex therapists. They clearly work, or else therapists would stop sending their clients off with them as homework.

The Sensate Focus Program has been around forever. It was standard practice for couples who'd lost a sexual connection right back when I wrote my first-ever book in 1999. I didn't include it and it doesn't feature prominently in any of my other books. The reason why is I didn't get it.

If I had a sex drought and wanted to break it, I'd be more likely to go away for the weekend, drink buckets of wine, and just do it rather than lie around stroking. The sex would probably be both basic and awkward, but at least I'd have done it and broken the drought, and then we could both go from there, introducing some exciting new stuff that's a bit edgy later on. For some couples, this may still be the best way to approach it.

Now that I'm older and calmer and (a little, not much) more patient, I realize that focusing on the mechanics of sex and not enough on the emotional side doesn't always work. Resurrecting your sex life might not just be about giving lust a rude prod and saying, "Wake up, you lazy bugger!" Lust needs bedfellows to work long-term. It needs togetherness and closeness as companions. Eroticism is an essential part of good sex, but you can't skip straight to that part—if you haven't been having regular sex—without re-laying the foundations.

Right now, you're both vulnerable. The gentleness of these programs might be just what you need.

THE WORLD'S EASIEST SEX PRACTICE

The first is by sex therapist Stephen Snyder, and it's called the Two-Step Plan. Now, read this carefully: the aim here is to experience arousal for arousal's sake. Not to have sex. Don't force it, and be patient. "Too many couples assume that every time they get aroused, they have to extinguish it with an orgasm—as if arousal was something irritating or unpleasant that has to be got rid of right away," Snyder says. (Oops! Definitely been guilty of that one!) Instead, he advises couples to experience their own arousal as something warm and nourishing. To let that feeling stay, live with it, before acting on it.

Snyder calls it "the world's easiest sex practice" because it really is.

Here's how to do it.

Step one: Lie in bed and do nothing. Get naked if you'd like to; if not, don't. Talk. It can be about anything but keep it simple: just enjoy lying beside each other with no agenda. Or just lie quietly and notice your breathing. You might like to stroke your partner's skin or your own. Keep the touching nonsexual at this point. Do it for as long as you're enjoying it. "You will feel awkward to start," says Snyder. "That's OK. Just acknowledge it, then let it go."

Step two: If you got aroused in step one, just enjoy the feeling. Don't feel you have to do anything with it. "Don't worry about arousal," Snyder says. "Let your arousal take care of you. Be a passenger and let it take you wherever it wants."

If it takes you to a place where you both decide you do want to have some type of sexual stimulation, go for it. Otherwise, hold on to the stillness and intimacy, says Snyder, and enjoy the moment. Get used to being naked together and aroused together.

And . . . that's it! Do this once a week for a month or two and then take it further if you want to.

This is a great technique for any couple to use, if you want to hit refresh and take sex back to basics again. Think of it as a sex detox as well as a gentle way to ease back into being erotic.

THE SENSATE FOCUS PROGRAM

Couples used to really like doing the Sensate Focus Program "maybe because it gave them a break from the terrible sex they were having," says Snyder wryly. Sensate Focus basically involves getting naked and taking turns caressing each other. Nonerotic to start with, then moving on to include erogenous zones and the genitals. You advance slowly: progressing from nonsexual to sexual touching could take weeks or months, not days.

The concept is simple: the person whose turn it is to touch focuses purely on doing just that. The recipient simply allows them to do it. The beauty of it, says Snyder, was that nobody had to worry about or take care of anyone else. You could relax.

He says couples these days aren't as enthusiastic. We have shorter attention spans and are more competitive. We try to come up with ways to be the best toucher ever and expect congratulations for our efforts. Fingers are itching to take selfies and Instagram the moment: #intimacy #connectingtime.

Programs like Sensate Focus and Two-Step are really about mindfulness. Paying attention without judgment and being in the present moment. Something we find increasingly hard to do in today's technology-based world, but really should master.

WHAT NEXT?

After you've worked through either the Two-Step Plan or Sensate Focus Program, work on breaking down the "chasing dynamic," says sex educator Emily Nagoski.

She recommends you take turns initiating sensual touching. Each person initiates at least once a week or every two weeks. It doesn't matter how often, so long as initiation is shared and neither feels pressured or deprived. From there, move on to simultaneous touching—touching each other sensually at the same time—then take the plunge, literally (if that's the aim), when ready. This might take weeks or months. No rush. Take your time.

FLIP THE SWITCH

As well as doing the physical exercises, work on changing your headspace. Instead of thinking, *I don't like sex anymore*, think: *How would I think if I were a woman or man who loved sex?*

Connect it to your identity, advises Nagoski. "Don't just run, be a runner. Don't just have sex, be a deliciously erotic person who is curious and playful about sex." Think: *If I were a person who loved sex, how would I deal with feeling too busy/sad/ tired/lonely for sex?*

"Pose your problem to that person. Let them solve it. I wonder what it would take for me to go from someone who dreads sex to someone who wants to jump my partner's bones?"

WHEN YOU DON'T WANT TO HAVE SEX ANYMORE

If you don't want sex but want to reignite desire with your partner, I'd suggest trying the Two-Step Plan or Sensate Focus Program (above) as well as reading chapter 5, which has lots of suggestions (they're peppered throughout the whole of the book, too).

If you're single and have decided sex is something you no longer need in your life, it's usually a matter of refusing to feel less than worthy just because you're not sexual anymore. Celibacy is on the rise and you have plenty of companions. Finding a partner who is also happy to be celibate, if you still want to find romance, is doable. Though it's an easier task the older you are.

This is for women who've decided they don't want to have sex again—ever—with their partner and want to know where to go from here.

As with your partner withdrawing sex, the reason why you've decided to stop will strongly dictate how well this news will be taken. If you can't bear to have sex with your partner again because there are severe relationship issues, this is very different than loving them and not wanting to be sexual. If that's the case— the relationship is so bad, you don't want physical contact of any sort—you have three choices. Confront your partner and attempt to talk things through, get therapy, or leave.

But there are plenty of you who will be reading this thinking, *No! I desperately love my partner. I'm just over the whole sex thing!* You want the man (or woman, depending on your sexual orientation) and you love your relationship, you just don't want the sex part. It happens, as I said.

Whatever the reason, if you want your partner to understand and work with you on this, you have to at least have made some attempt to solve the problem. Things like going to see a doctor or gynecologist if painful sex is the issue, trying some of the suggestions in this book in an attempt to spark some interest, or thinking about why sex has never really appealed to you, if that's the case. When they ask, "Have you tried to fix this?" you need to be able to say yes and mean it.

Define what you mean by "no sex"

My next question is: would you consider nonreciprocal sex with your partner? Lots of women say they don't want sex, but what they mean is they don't want intercourse or penetrative sex.

Would you be happy having foreplay? If you're not interested in being sexually stimulated yourself, would you be happy doing something to your partner (like oral sex, hand jobs, etc.)? What about lying beside them as they masturbate? If you think you could be sexual, but just don't want sex the way it looks now, say so. Be honest and you might be pleasantly surprised.

You don't want to do anything sexual at all? If you're in a monogamous relationship and your partner's not done with sex, that leaves them in a very unfortunate situation. Sex for them now means solo sex sessions, fantasizing, and watching porn. For some people, this will be enough. Especially if your reason for wanting to stop is because of something outside your control, like a health issue. If, instead, it's a choice, it's a different scenario. You're basically saying to your partner: I want you to be sexually faithful to me, but I won't have sex with you.

Does this seem fair to you?

Every couple's circumstances are different and you may well be justified in saying, "Actually, yes it does, given what's happened." But, even if you do think it's fair, be aware that your relationship is now at risk. If you're not having sex with your partner and your partner's dying for it, everyone around them is going to look mighty appealing. Even if they are the most loyal partner on the planet and love you dearly, there is a chance they will succumb to temptation if someone else pays them attention. Or they might decide to use sex workers on a regular basis. This is a popular option for men who love their partner but still desire sex. They figure there's no (or low) risk they'll fall in love, so it feels less like cheating, and discretion is assured.

You have several choices about how to deal with this:

Accept that your partner might have an affair. You hope like hell they won't but are prepared to take the risk of them seeking unapproved sex outside the relationship.

Hint that you would understand if they got sex elsewhere without officially giving permission. By this, I mean allude to it: "I know this makes it difficult for you, and I understand you need to do what you need to do."

Maybe we need to learn to think outside the box. We have no problem saying, "I'm not going to the theater again because I can't sit for that long with my arthritic hips. I know you're still passionate about it, why don't you go with a friend?"

Relax the rules of monogamy. This might mean you allow your partner to have sex with other people, with your permission. If that's something you think you could do, think about how this might work. As I said earlier, couples who agree to do it usually have strict rules—like it can't be someone you know, no repeats, etc. Sometimes people want to know; others give permission and never want to know. Whatever happens, if you allow your partner to get their needs met elsewhere, it has to happen respectfully and safely. If you agree to be polyamorous (allow them to have romantic relationships as well as sex), it's even more important to set rules.

Separate or divorce. Sometimes, having this conversation ends the relationship. "I told my husband of 40 years I no longer wanted to be sexual with him, and he sat me down, held my hands, looked me in the eye, and said, 'I'm so sorry but I can't stay with you knowing that. It would break my heart.' We separated and are now divorced. Do I regret it? No. I am happier single and not being hassled, and we're still good friends." Other stories don't end as happily.

All of these factors need much thought before you say to your partner, "Hey, you know sex? Well, I'm not doing that anymore." It's one hell of a statement.

AFFAIRS:
YOURS, THEIRS,
=== AND ===

DEALING

 # FALLOUT

TWENTY YEARS AGO, ANYTHING WRITTEN or said about infidelity was almost certainly from the victim's perspective. Cheaters were bad people and were going to hell for it, and God help anyone who dared to suggest otherwise.

Then a funny thing happened. Research suggested it wasn't just bad people who were cheating—nice people were at it as well. Even more alarming was that people in happy relationships who loved their partners and had no problems were also doing it.

Hang on a minute! Don't people seek sex elsewhere when their wives don't understand them and they aren't getting any at home? The final nail in the coffin of old perceptions of why people are unfaithful: women now do it (almost) as much as men do. The end result of all these new discoveries is that there are some damn interesting conversations being had about the nature of infidelity—mainly by women, interestingly—and fresh, new ways of looking at it.

Esther Perel's TED Talk "Why Happy Couples Cheat" has been viewed millions of times; her previous TED Talk "Rethinking Infidelity" had more than four million views at the time of writing. The reason why I quote her extensively in this chapter is that no one has wrestled with the topic and tried to understand it more than Perel. Except, perhaps, biological anthropologist Helen Fisher. Her classic text, *Anatomy of Love: A Natural History of Mating, Marriage, and Why We Stray*, was recently updated and republished after more than 20 years. US sex and couples therapist Dr. Tammy Nelson's recent book is titled *When You're the One Who Cheats: Ten Things You Need to Know*. Cheating is a hot topic.

Fisher estimates that 40 percent of us cheat, one US study said 50 percent of women cheat, and Perel puts it at anything between

26 and 75 percent because there is no universally agreed-upon definition of what constitutes an infidelity in our digital age.

Technology makes it easier to sneak illicit sex but—be warned—it's also harder to hide. The old lipstick on the collar and suspicious receipts could be got around. Discovery today comes via a default setting that helpfully syncs all your devices so that texts from your mistress appear on the kids' iPads just as your wife's helping them with their homework.

WHY ARE WE ALL AT IT?

Let me count the ways. Nelson thinks men cheat for companionship and intimacy—if it's just sex that's lacking, they turn to porn. If love and affection are lacking, they have an affair. Women, she says, cheat for passion and sex—erotic sex. We're tired of looking after our men and want selfish sex without complications.

Many women are serial cheaters, according to Wednesday Martin, the author of *Untrue*, a book that overturns the stereotype that says men are more sexual than women. We marry the boring guy because he's stable and reliable and would make a great dad, then have steamy sex on the side with the hot, bad ones. That way we get the security, stability, and companionship of long-term love but the excitement of erotic sex.

Fisher cites research that shows 34 percent of women and 56 percent of men who have had affairs describe their marriage as happy or very happy. "From a Darwinian perspective, we were probably evolved to want it all," Fisher says. "And now we live in a stage of human evolution where we can actually get it all."

US sex therapist Stephen Snyder maintains our "sexual self"—something within us that operates by its own distinct set of rules—behaves like a child. "Your sexual self doesn't understand the whole monogamy thing. Sometimes it just wants what it wants, and there's no reasoning with it," he writes. "If you're like most people, your sexual self would love to have it both ways. It likes the security of being exclusive, but once in a while it wouldn't mind some action on the side."

Which is why reading this bit—the reasons why *you* might succumb to the call of the wild—all sounds, well, quite logical and oddly innocent, really. It's when you're on the *other* end of infidelity and the ground's pulled out from under you that the flip side emerges.

When affairs are discovered, the fallout is usually catastrophic. The person having the affair knows it's possible to love two people, while the person who's been loving just one, wholeheartedly, feels duped and devastated.

Don't ever kid yourself that what you're doing is OK just because everyone's doing it. When you're standing in front of someone you love dearly, who is holding your phone in their hands and looking at you in horrified bewilderment, what you did is all that matters.

Why men cheat

Men's reasons are much the same as women's. He might have an affair for excitement, if he's bored or disappointed with his life (someone else gets that longed-for promotion). Or he meets an old friend who's now fat and aging, then looks in the mirror and sees double. There's nothing like an affair to give you an ego boost and make you feel better about yourself.

Mistresses idolize—they see the reflection in the pond. A wife sees the true him—under a microscope. Not too many wives idealize their husbands, but a lot of men love to be hero-worshipped.

Affairs are all about pinpoint focus: you become the only two people in the world. Reality recedes and it's flattering as hell. This is also why the minute an affair comes out into the open, most shrivel and die. You simply can't maintain that focus 24/7 and live your life.

The other reason men cheat is for sex. If you're withholding sex from a long-term partner, the chances of him having an affair increase substantially. This is a risk you take when you decide to end your sexual relationship with your partner (and one I discuss in detail in chapter 5).

Some men think they'll cheat just once, if in a sexless marriage, then realize just how much they wanted sex and needed sex, so they don't stop doing it. Perel says those who are unfaithful are often people who have been faithful for decades but one day cross a line they never thought they would cross.

Tempted?

Listen, good people cheat. I've made that clear. You're not a monster for wanting to or even for following through. But if you intend to turn cheating into a lifestyle choice, don't gloss over what you're doing. If your partner wouldn't be fazed, consider suggesting an open relationship. If they would and you love them, can you handle living with the guilt and deception?

If the answer to that is no and you're considering sex with someone other than your partner, but you want to keep them, don't trivialize what you're contemplating. Instead, set limits. Say no to yourself, don't wrestle with what-ifs. Don't have the private dinner with that sexy work colleague on a business trip. Don't go for office drinks if you know you'll flirt. Remove temptation.

Recognize how dangerous serious flirtation is. Longing is a powerful emotion. If there's someone who has ignited that in you, don't give it oxygen. Don't tease and banter, don't hint that you're not entirely happy at home. Don't think "just once" will be enough. Set boundaries and don't cross them.

Most crucially, turn toward your partner, not away, and work on trying to find the element you're craving with them. If you're at the drowning, not waving, stage and need to shock them to take you seriously, admit you were tempted to have an affair. It's risky, sure, but you didn't act on it, and if this doesn't get their attention, it's time for divorce, not therapy.

IT'S NOT YOU, IT'S ME

It really is, in lots of cases. Here are 11 reasons why your partner cheating had nothing to do with you or your relationship.

1. Serial adulterers can't do intimacy. It doesn't matter who they end up with, they will always cheat because the alternative is to get too close to someone. This must be avoided at all costs because they might get hurt.

2. They've got other issues. Affairs are a great way to distract yourself from painful feelings you've never resolved.

3. They want to feel young again. Sneaking around, being "naughty": affairs remind us of being young. They want to recapture parts of themselves that have been lost as well as check they've still "got it."

4. They want sexual intensity, which can't be maintained long-term. No matter how good a lover you are, you can't replicate the erotic potency that sleeping with someone new brings.

5. They're mourning missed opportunities. What if they'd chosen another path? What if they'd taken up other romantic opportunities? Having an affair now could be them playing out the past.

6. They don't like who they've become. Perel, as usual, puts it perfectly: "When we seek the gaze of another, it isn't always our partner that we are turning away from, but the person that we have ourselves become. And it isn't so much that we're looking for another person, as much as we are looking for another self."

7. They want freedom. If they've been happily married for years but got together young, the affair could be their chance to explore the freedom they missed out on.

8. It's in their genes. A Swedish study of 552 men suggested infidelity could be partly genetic: it's in our DNA.

9. It's a way of dealing with life's transitions. Turning a certain age, retiring, kids leaving home. Not liking where you're at and wanting some excitement—all are common reasons people cite as motivation.

10. They're an antidote to death. "All over the world, there is one word that people who have affairs always tell me. They feel alive," Perel says. "And they will often tell me stories of recent losses—a parent who died, a friend that went too soon, and bad news at the doctor." It's not uncommon for people who lose someone dear to them to suddenly want sex. Sex, after all, is how we create life. It appeals on a deep, psychological level.

11. Because it's entirely possible to love and lust after more than one person at once. Fisher says we've evolved three distinctly different brain systems for mating and reproduction: the sex drive, feelings of intense romantic love, and deep attachment to a long-term partner. These three brain systems are often very well connected, she says, but not always: "You can lie in bed at night and feel deep attachment to a long-term partner, and then your brain can swing into feelings of wild, romantic love for somebody else, and then your brain can swing into feelings of the sex drive for people that you hardly know, in the office or social circle."

HOW TO HEAL AFTER INFIDELITY

Here's the deal: sometimes you *shouldn't* try to repair the damage and try to forgive. If your relationship is hanging by a thread, your partner treats you badly, or love left a long time ago, why on earth would you try to forgive if you discover they've been unfaithful? Take it as the death knell it is. Get the hell out of there and direct your energy toward separating and creating a new life for yourself.

Similarly, if this isn't the first affair you've discovered, and the last hurt you badly, follow the "three strikes and you're out" rule. If your partner saw you go through agony and then went right back out that door and did it again, don't kid yourself. This is going to be your life if you stay. (If you are kidding yourself, take yourself off to a tough-love therapist and let them talk sense into you.)

It's still worth reading the rest of the chapter; even if you split, you still need to make sense of things so you can trust again and find peace. Just don't waste more time on a relationship that isn't worth another second of it.

But what if your relationship is great, you are best friends with your partner, you both love your kids, sex wasn't amazing but it wasn't bad either, and then you discover your partner's been unfaithful? What next? The betrayal feels even worse if you're in a good relationship. Or what if it's you who strayed and you're standing in the middle of the train wreck that used to be your life, knowing you're the one who caused all the pain and anguish?

When one of you has just made the discovery, the betrayal can feel so traumatic and shattering, it feels like no one could survive it. But once the pain subsides—and it will—you might think differently. The fact is, the majority of couples who have experienced affairs stay together. If your relationship is worth fighting for, fight for it. Here's what the journey from hell back to happiness might look like.

What happens to sex and love after an affair

Dr. Tammy Nelson believes most couples pass through three stages of recovery, if they are to recover:

1. THE CRISIS PHASE

Once the affair is discovered, depending on your coping mechanisms and personality, you'll either be heavily sedated and in a dark room or smashing up anything your partner holds dear. Emotional instability, sleeplessness, angry arguments, uncontrollable sobbing, extreme anger or intense sadness, feeling like you won't survive the pain, confusion, bewilderment, hatred, and fear of being left and alone—you will experience any or all of these emotions.

Some couples separate and the deceived person refuses to see their partner until the pain eases. Or the person feels so much anger and pain they can't bear the thought of their partner touching them. Others do the opposite and cling on tight. "My partner had a text affair with an old friend. He got a little bit of attention from another female and he thought it was OK to pursue it. I found out, and it stopped. It did affect our sex life but in a better way. He desired me more, not less. Like he didn't want to let go. It was the thought that he could have lost me. I felt confused at the time, but I did feel desired, which gave me my confidence back."

Lots of couples find they're having more sex with each other post-affair than ever before—passionate, intense sex, says Nelson. There are several reasons why this happens. First, you desperately want to connect because you're terrified you'll lose each other. Second, primal "mate guarding" kicks in: you want to lay claim to what's yours. Third, the affair creates distance between you—and distance fuels desire.

It's the close couples, remember, that experience desire problems. Who is this person? You thought you knew your partner, but you don't. Desire is reborn, says Nelson, because you're effectively sleeping with a new person and our bodies love novelty. You also see your partner through the other person's eyes. When someone else wants what we have, things become far more attractive: you appreciate what you didn't before.

Even if you hate yourself for having wild, fantastic sex—you don't want your partner to think you've forgiven them—it happens. Or it doesn't. Both reactions are normal.

"I wanted to have sex with him but every time he touched me, I saw his hands touching her. How could I ever have sex with him again?"

2. THE INSIGHT PHASE

This is when there's less blame and more curiosity, says Nelson. The focus shifts from what the sex was like to the emotions felt.

This is the time to get couples therapy, she advises. You're both more logical and thinking more clearly—though that's not to say it's any less painful. "You don't need to forgive at this point," Nelson warns. "It's too soon. You'll take it back again." Instead, aim for empathy: try to understand what it's been like to live in each other's worlds. "Instead of a good person and a bad person, you realize you each share responsibility for at least part of what happened." It's more "How did this happen to us?" than "You heartless bitch/bastard, I hope you rot in hell."

It might be rude, but it is a wake-up call to the fact that relationships need nurturing and attention. That your partner won't just hang around if you only feed them crumbs. That sex is important, and they aren't immune to other people's charms. In short, an affair can provide the kick in the pants both of you needed.

3. THE VISION PHASE

Affairs either signal the end or a new beginning.

"My wife had me on the shortest leash you could imagine: she was pathologically jealous and would fly off the handle at anything. I lived like that for 12 years, not going anywhere or doing anything that might upset her, and then turned 50 and thought: I'm living my life before it's over. The affair was part of that. It was with a work colleague and didn't last long but my wife found out and it turned us around. She realized she could no longer control me and had no option but to trust. I guess the thing she feared the most—me being unfaithful—happened and she survived. She finally relaxed and we are very happy. If the affair hadn't been discovered and things continued the way they were, I'd have left."

It's during the vision phase that you see possibilities rather than problems. This is when you decide if you want to stay together and create a new future—one that satisfies both of you. The memory of the third person disappears, says Nelson, when you have new experiences together and do new things.

Good things can come out of affairs—and the person who often ends up benefiting is the deceived partner. "You think I didn't want more?" is the common, thunderous reaction of the wronged party, Perel says. Once the affair is exposed, they no longer have to pretend they're completely satisfied and happy, either with mediocre sex or zero attention. If your partner's in the doghouse, you get to call the shots.

In the aftermath of an affair, couples "will have depths of conversation with honesty and openness that they haven't had in decades. And partners who were sexually indifferent find themselves suddenly so lustfully voracious, they don't know where it's coming from," Perel says.

If you get through to the other side, many couples fall in love all over again—but ignore the erotic side of your relationship at your peril. You need love and sex to survive: lots of affairs happen because, while love grows, sex is allowed to wither and die.

Excuse me, but that's so not happening to us

So, that's the path some couples take to get to the other side. I would suggest these are couples that are good communicators, have a strong foundation of love and respect, and are both emotionally strong enough to cope with the shock of an affair. Which means there are a lot of you stuck at the darkest part, with not even a glimmer of light at the end of the tunnel.

If this is you, remember that recovery is not a straight line. One day you'll think you're through it, both laughing and swigging back wine like you used to, and then suddenly you'll remember and both be thrown back into the bitterness of day one of discovery with a force that knocks you over again. Some couples take years before they get back to normal. UK sex therapist Andrew Marshall has written lots about infidelity and warns that full confession can take months and months: highly frustrating for the person who is trying to understand why someone who loves them has caused them such pain.

If you don't know how to react or what to do with the hurt and can't move forward, find a good therapist. They are trained to help you both sort through the myriad emotions you're experiencing. Most of all, don't feel pressure to forgive and don't even try to forget. It takes time. If your partner tries to hurry you along, remind them that they're the reason you're in this place.

A psychiatrist once told me our tendency to want to rush to find solutions means we often make the wrong decision. However uncomfortable it feels, the longer you stay at the point of indecision, the better decision you will make. If you aren't sure if the relationship is worth saving, stay still until you are sure.

Doing this will help you move forward

Every couple deals with an affair differently, but certain things help everyone. All these tips apply to both sexes; they are, instead, distinguished by who had the affair.

IF *THEY* HAD THE AFFAIR

Don't make any long-term decisions at the start. If you can't stand to have your partner in the house, by all means throw them out until the anger is manageable. Just don't do anything that you can't undo at this point.

Ask if they practiced safe sex. If they didn't or you don't believe they did, ask your doctor to check for sexually transmitted diseases (STDs) and HIV.

It's normal to feel overwhelmed with grief. You are grieving the end of a relationship you trusted and the rosy future you thought you had.

This is the first era in which there's more shame in staying after an affair than leaving, says Perel. "Rather than appreciating the maturity, courage, and tenacity that it takes to stay in a relationship after this trauma and trying to improve it, we imagine it shows weak character."

Staying in a bad or abusive relationship after an affair is harmful. Trying to work through it when you're in a good relationship, especially if this behavior is completely out of character, is the right thing to do.

Cover yourself with a blanket of love from friends and family, and do things that give you joy. It's important to reaffirm your sense of self-worth and remind yourself of the strong, confident you that's still there, just MIA.

Don't ask for sordid details, "questions that only inflict pain and keep you awake at night," Perel advises. She tells the story of a woman who found out about her husband's affair and "went digging." She found "hundreds of messages and photos exchanged and desires expressed. Affairs in the digital age are death by a thousand cuts."

Skip the "I bet they were thinner/sexier/better in bed than me" and instead ask "investigative" questions like, "What did the affair mean to you?"

The hardest thing to get over is that you lose the "we." If you're close and do everything together, the fact that your partner went off and had an "adventure" without you, hurts almost as much as the infidelity.

Betrayal destroys the idea that one person can be everything to another—that it's the two of you against the world. It's like finding out Santa doesn't exist at the age of three, multiplied by a billion. "Betrayal steals the story of your life," Perel says. No wonder you're on your knees.

The second hardest is this: as much as your partner might regret hurting you, they may not regret having had the affair. Your brain and your heart will both explode when first hearing them say these words. But hang in there, it might make sense later on.

Even if the affair wasn't about sex, it feels like it's about sex because sex is the most intimate thing you do with your partner. Sex can be the Achilles' heel of an otherwise strong relationship, says Marshall. "Time and time again, I see couples who are really good friends, really good at sorting stuff, but they've never managed to sort sex out. Affairs are not all about sex, but sex is often a large part."

At some point, sex has to become part of your relationship again or you will forever just be friends. Have brutally honest conversations about what you both want sexually and don't be scared to criticize your old selves. This is a new relationship—make new rules!

Take baby steps. You will feel angry when you first become intimate. Even if you went through the shagging-like-rabbits post-affair stage, there will come a time when sex makes you angry or cry. The ghost of the other person is there for both of you, and time and patience are the only things that work to drive them out of your bed and your head.

Start by simply cuddling, then progress from there. Don't give up even if lots of sessions end with you storming off or in tears. The Sensate Focus Program or Two-Step Plan might work for you (see page 202). See a sex therapist if you feel you aren't progressing at all and don't forget afterplay. Cuddle, chat, lie there together— it's just as important.

Don't use the affair to win every argument, says Marshall, even if you can and even though it's so tempting, years and years later.

Make time for your partner. "He was always at work, on his phone, doing things—everything was important except for me," said one woman. "He said afterward, he did everything *for* me. But I didn't care about the big house, I just wanted time with him and I never got it."

"Affairs are way less about sex and a lot more about desire: desire for attention, desire to feel special, desire to feel important," says Perel. Make your partner feel all these things: make sure they do the same for you.

Own your part in it. Of course you aren't to blame for your partner having an affair, but it takes two to make a problem. Take responsibility for your part.

"There are many ways that we betray our partner: with contempt, with neglect, with indifference, with violence. Sexual betrayal is only one way to hurt a partner. In other words, the victim of an affair is not always the victim of the marriage," Perel wisely says.

What do you regret? Not making time for your partner? Always rejecting sex? Not giving compliments? Not saying "I love you"? Continue to make the same mistakes and your relationship will end up back in the same place.

IF *YOU* HAD THE AFFAIR

Admit that you fucked up. Because you really did. Even if the affair was the best thing that ever happened to you, even if you think your partner drove you to it, you have to acknowledge the pain it's caused. Later, you can talk about some of the reasons that contributed to you straying, but you must never forget that you hurt someone who loved you by choosing to have an affair.

Make your partner feel safe. You're here with them now. You know you hurt them badly and you're truly sorry.

The lying does as much damage as the cheating. Honesty is the basis of all good relationships. It takes years to rebuild trust, if indeed it can be rebuilt. Apart from social lies, you cannot lie about anything from here on.

Honesty is essential but tact even more so. It's obvious the type of questions your partner is likely to ask. Think about how you'll reply.

If you were the one who cheated, it is not going to help matters to answer "Was he better than me in bed?" with: "Yes. Amazing actually. I'd always wondered what it was like to sleep with a man with a really large penis." Hearing, "It was someone new. The novelty made it exciting" is easier to stomach.

What did you get from the affair that you weren't getting from your partner? The first thing a good therapist will do is ask who you were in the affair: what sort of person were you in that relationship compared to the person you are with your partner?

Think about how you could fulfill those needs with your partner. Be clear about what you want and need from them—when you're at the fixing stage. (Presenting them with a list as long as your arm two weeks after they found out will simply get you a divorce.)

You must now be totally transparent. This means your partner knows all the passwords to everything, the code to your phone. The lot. Some people won't want that, but others will demand it, at least for a while. You can't blame them. Besides, if you're going to keep your nose clean, what will there be for them to find?

Healing comes from small daily acts of kindness, rather than grand gestures. Making a cup of tea. Saying "I love you." Going out of your way to pick your partner up, make their day better. (Throwing in the odd trip to Paris won't go astray either.)

Your partner shouldn't have to ask for information or reassurance. If you cheated with someone from work, come home and immediately let them know if you had contact with the person. How you felt nothing, how they have nothing to worry about.

What if they do have something to worry about and you're tempted to have another affair or continue it? The decent thing to do is to let them know you no longer want to be monogamous or you want to be with the person you had the affair with. The really shitty thing to do is to pretend it's all over and continue to see them or start something up with someone else. You're not that kind of person, surely?

FIFTY-SOMETHING
AND
SINGLE

THE NUMBER OF "SILVER SINGLES"—people over 50 out there dating again after decades in a relationship—is rising. Partners die, or leave, or we do the same: it's life.

Unfortunately, it's life for women more so than men. Statistically, women are far more likely to be widowed and far less likely to remarry than men. We make up 11 million of the 13 million bereaved spouses in the US, and the number of widowed females in Australia is significantly higher than men.

In an age when divorce is less common for younger people, the divorce rate for American adults aged 50 and older has roughly doubled since the 1990s. In 2017, the number of divorces in the UK was highest among both men and women aged 45 to 49 years. "Gray divorce" (I'm sensing a theme here) is being led by Baby Boomers. This is because there were unprecedented levels of divorce when we were young, making us less sure our own marriages would last. We're more likely to be on our second (third, fourth) marriage approaching 50, making divorce more likely after it. Statistics vary on whether second or later marriages last, but if you've divorced once, it's far less scary to do it again. Recent American statistics show the divorce rate for adults post-50 who have married before is double the rate of those who've only been married once.

Happy days, eh? Let me lift your spirits a little.

BEING SINGLE CAN BE LIBERATING

Not all women mourn the departure of their partner. Lots are more than happy to wave them off. *The Merry Widow* might be the name of an opera, but it also encapsulates how a lot of women feel, finally free after enduring a stifling, banal marriage or relationship with a controlling, demanding partner who made life joyless.

Of course, there are women who are left bereft and desperately unhappy after death or divorce, but equally as many aren't interested in finding another long-term partner. Lots feel perfectly happy (or happier) on their own and/or are only interested in short-term flings, if and when they happen.

Even if you don't want to stay solo, being single again offers a chance to start over: to find someone who is compatible with who you are now, rather than who you were. *Eat, Pray, Love* author Elizabeth Gilbert, Cynthia Nixon (Miranda in *Sex and the City*), and Portia de Rossi (*Ally McBeal* and *Arrested Development*) well and truly wiped the slate clean by swapping men for women. We care less what other people think when we're older and time becomes finite. These are good things.

Whatever category you fall into, being single post-50 is different than being single in the first half of your life. Instead of meeting at a disco or pub, you'll be scrolling through pages of potential partner "résumés" on dating apps. The three-date rule has become the your-choice rule; sexually transmitted diseases aren't just loitering around, they're on the rise; and the younger men you'd eye off with an "I wish" while partnered up might just be your new date. Good job! I'm here to take you through it all, having navigated all this myself!

HOW DO WOMEN FEEL ABOUT BEING SINGLE AND OVER 50?

This is what women told me about their experience of being single.

"I'm one of an ever-growing group! The postmortgage, postdivorce crowd. Women are more independent than ever, me included. I've always worked and was told never to rely on a man— by my dad, who actually was the most reliable man in the world. But I miss having someone there for the simple stuff: sharing decisions, sharing costs, going on holidays, and Christmas."

"I had quite a good marriage, but now I'm single. He cheated, and I wish I'd left ages ago. I'm having the time of my life. I had my first oral sex orgasm a month ago. My husband never went down on me."

"I'm single for life, I think! All the men of my age look so much older than me and have no appeal. All the younger guys who are hot are not going to be interested in a dried-up old bird!"

"I've always been perfectly happy with short-term relationships and made the most of being single. But now I want to settle down; I'm lonely. I'm good at being single but it's hard now. I'm more home focused. I want someone to watch TV with and go on holiday with."

"You should never rely on anyone else to make you happy, it's up to you. I'm not a 'be with anyone rather than be alone' kind of person."

"I'm way more confident this time around. I forgive my body for its flaws now. It's made an enormous difference to sex."

"The trick is to find other friends who are also single. If you have a few friends to go out with, being single can be a real laugh. I'm in no hurry to fall into another long-term relationship. I'm very happy playing the field. It's different now than it was because there are lots of single people over 50 out there."

"I was with my husband from the age of 16 to my mid-fifties, then he died. I'm now 60. It's been a huge paradigm shift to get used to doing things alone when we did everything as a couple. I miss the sex most of all. I'm not enjoying being single—I'm not desperate, but I'm lonely."

"I thought I'd grow old with my husband. That wasn't in the cards for us. But maybe it's in the cards for me with someone else."

"I'm incredibly lonely but scared to death to even try to meet someone because I have put on weight since menopause and suffer from vaginal dryness and constant UTIs."

"I'd like a part-time relationship where we enhanced each other's lives rather than become their life. This is common in older guys who are retired and have a lot of time to fill."

"I'm having the time of my life. Try a younger man. You'll never go back to the oldies!"

"I'd rather be single than be with an idiot."

HOW TO FIND A PARTNER POST-50

I was single creeping up to 50 and I know what it's like—fantastic at times, bloody awful at others. My constant lament was "Why are there so many older women who are attractive, bright, kind, clever, and single—and no male equivalents?" Any single guy I met around my own age had a big "reject" stamp on his head: it was clear within a month of seeing them why they hadn't been snapped up.

I dated the sweet guy who quickly revealed himself to be an alcoholic. I dated the handsome guy who had (scary) anger issues. I dated the tall guy who was attached to his mother by rope, not apron strings (even more frightening). The reason I went out with them, even though I suspected their flaws before they became screamingly obvious, was because there weren't any other options.

I used to meet at least one new woman I liked and admired every week. I've met one fantastic single man in the last decade and I'm now married to him.

Don't head for the cliff just yet though: you only need one person, after all (well, assuming you're not into polyamory). At least six of my previously single friends also happened to meet one fantastic single man, after looking for years, and are also happily coupled up. They are out there but, Jesus, you need confidence, determination, and an excellent sense of humor to find the bastards.

In search of the elusive single man

Where are they? All the single men over 50 who are intelligent, attractive, solvent, and sane? They can't all be dead or gay. Are they hiding in that rundown pub you walk past and never go into? At home watching Netflix? At their computer watching porn only to emerge for food supplies?

Why don't they go out like women do, preferably all together so you get a choice? The only time I ever see a group of middle-aged men, they're on a cheap flight on the way to Prague for a stag night. And nine out of 10 of them have wedding rings on.

Dateable men over 50 are like species on the borderline of extinction: occasionally sighted and with much excitement when they are. Or are they out there, among us, and we're simply not noticing them?

A psychotherapist friend once said to me that all middle-aged men look the same and it's only when you get to know them that they become attractive. Think of three men your own age that you already know, who you'd date if they were single or you are really, really fond of, and you might just find she's right. Imagine seeing a picture of them on a dating app, without knowing their personality. Would you click or swipe right? There's a lesson to be learned there.

FOUR GOOD PRINCIPLES TO GO BY

I can think of many, but as I have to narrow it down (so you're not reading a book of a billion pages), I vote for these.

Focus on the things that matter

Height doesn't matter. His bank balance doesn't matter (unless he has real money issues like gambling or living way beyond his means, in which case it most certainly does). Clothes sense really doesn't matter (most men are happy to be styled if necessary). His job doesn't matter, especially if he really loves doing it.

There needs to be some sexual attraction, but that doesn't mean they have to be good-looking. Charisma trumps chiseled cheekbones or a square jaw any day.

Kindness is critical. Niceness also. Being able to love you the way you want to be loved is essential (and something you only find out over time). Respect is paramount. Making a big effort with your family and kids is another must. Thinking you're the sexiest thing they've seen in years is vital if you want a good sexual relationship. Sexual technique isn't important because it can be taught.

All this applies regardless of sexual orientation.

You'll also have your own list of absolute musts—just make sure they're musts that matter.

Go younger

"I'm trying to wean myself off younger men," was the headline of an article in the *Observer* about me when I was in my late forties. I wasn't lying: I'd get older, but the age of my boyfriends remained the same. Between 10 or even 20 years younger than me.

You already know one reason why—I didn't meet any men my own age that I was interested in. But I did meet lots of younger guys who not only looked great and had the energy and outlook I found attractive, but they also found *me* attractive. "Men my own age either find me threatening (alpha males and I have always clashed) or want younger models, even though I look young for my age," one woman wrote to me. "I find it ironic that I can pull a good-looking 30-year-old at the age of 52, but not a very average 55-year-old man."

Another happy customer writes: "When I was 43, I dated a guy who was 23 and a few others who were under 30. Much more fun! They have a zest for life and take much more care of themselves." (More on why the older woman, younger man combination works on page 254.)

The perceived "man shortage" isn't helped by the fact that most women prefer men who are older than they are. It's hard-wired into us and also a choice because men who are older than us tend to be richer than us. When a young woman chooses an older man for this reason—money or evolution—she steals what men there are available for older women. Beat the system: go younger.

I'm not suggesting that you settle down with some guy who's a decade or so younger than you (though if you really like each other, why the hell not?), but I am saying broaden your horizons and not all relationships have to be long ones. A fling or two with someone younger could be just what you need to keep you amused or give you an ego boost. (For the record, I did wean myself off; my husband is a mere three years younger than me, which doesn't count.)

Do some navel gazing

Along with the "reject"-stamped dates, I did actually date some very nice men. I was the one who messed those relationships up.

I had a dreadful habit of asking other people's opinions about three dates in, before I'd really made up my mind about the person. Friends are protective and take the job of vetting seriously. They will point out faults you never saw before the poor guy's had the chance to reveal the really good aspects of himself that aren't immediately apparent, which might balance them out.

When I met Miles, my husband, I didn't introduce him to anyone for months, and when I did, I didn't ask their opinion because I already knew I really liked him. The other thing I did differently with Miles was admit I wanted a relationship.

I used to pretend I wasn't the "settle down" type, because it seemed much cooler to say that. (In my defense, I actually wasn't for about 20 years—I was way too career-oriented and having a ball—but I was keen to meet someone later on.) I was also aware I'd sabotage relationships. My dad had an affair when I was a teen and I had (major) trust issues. I was fine for a few months, but when I started to really fall for someone, I'd subconsciously sabotage it. I got some therapy over the years, but it still didn't stop me trying it with Miles. The difference was, when he called me on it, I recognized that's what I was doing and stopped.

The point of me telling you all this is that if I hadn't done lots of navel gazing and therapy to identify patterns of behavior that weren't working for me, I would still be single rather than incredibly happy, eight years into a relationship. Know yourself. Know your patterns. Ask your friends what mistakes they think you make, the wrong signals you send. Listen to them. Do things differently.

Don't force love

I know. When you're lonely and on your 30th date (or haven't had any at all for 30 months) and feeling down and desperate, it can feel like anyone is better than no one. If that means you relax rigid standards, this moment is a breakthrough. If it means you're going to make yourself pretend to love someone just because you want another live human in your house, I promise it won't work.

Nothing is lonelier than being in the wrong relationship. Get a dog or roommate instead.

DO I REALLY HAVE TO? DATING APPS AND ONLINE DATING

My 18-year-old stepdaughter thinks not going online or using an app to find a partner is odd. "It's counterintuitive," she says. "How else are you going to meet loads of people all at once? Old people see the same people all the time. How else would they meet some-one new?" she asks, genuinely baffled.

Very few people post-40 enjoy choosing a partner online or on an app. You're not alone in clinging to the old-fashioned notion of face-to-face communication, and you absolutely don't have to date using technology. But why wouldn't you use everything at your disposal?

It's 50/50 on whether technology will work for you

I would never advise anyone to pin all their hopes of finding a new partner on technology, because it works for some and not others. I know lots of people who've used apps or websites to find a part-ner. Roughly half have been successful and loved the process: they are the good-looking, socially gregarious ones who are also com-fortable with technology. The other half hated it and had mortify-ing, disastrous experiences—people who are shy, less photogenic, more sensitive.

You need a tough skin to survive apps and online dating. You need a sense of humor and good friends that you can call when you're left sitting there, waiting for a date who doesn't arrive. Or will call you to save you from dates who are dire when they do show.

But technology is a highly effective way to search for love or sex if you're after something specific, because there's an app or website for everyone. Love dancing and want to meet another dancer? There's an app for that. Want someone in uniform? Ditto. Think of virtually anything that's on your "must" list and you'll find it online somewhere. (Some of the big dating sites start niche websites and simply feed through people on theirs that have ticked the box you want. But hey, at least they've done the filtering for you!) Technology is also useful if it's hard for you to go out to meet people. Or if you live in a small town with few prospects and need to look further afield.

The way to use it effectively is to make it another string to your bow. Don't just join a dating website or download an app; go to singles events so you meet people in person as well. Ask your friends to set you up, keep your eye out when you're out with friends, talk to strangers if you find them attractive, look up not down when you're out and about and on public transport. Try everything, then decide what works for you. Usually, it's a combination of lots of things.

There's lots of information out there on which apps and websites are the most popular for which age group, how to join them, how to navigate them, and how to write a great profile online and choose photos that work for you. Do your research before joining.

Here are some other things to keep in mind.

Don't be conned. There are people out there who are out to get what they can. That might be no-strings sex (and if that's what you're also after, great!). It also might be your money.

If someone seems too good to be true, they generally are. If you've fallen for someone and they suddenly want money for an operation, a loan, anything you feel uncomfortable giving, get out of there. Watch *Dirty John* on Netflix if you think it won't happen to you. Some con men come in mightily attractive packages—that's how they get away with it.

Find the right site that works for you. Do your research. Ask friends. Experiment. Try at least a couple before giving up. Apps tend to suit younger people who are comfortable with dating, using technology, and who like more casual dates and relationships. Try a traditional dating website if you're not checking those boxes.

It takes a while for the average person to find someone. My friends all seemed to go through the same cycle: they'd join up, date like mad for about a month or two, get jaded, and take a break. Then go back online, be more discerning, and either end up meeting someone after a few dates or give up completely. Though I do know one woman who met her husband on the first date she had, the first time she ever went online.

Don't fall for expensive dating services. They don't work. I have three or four friends who forked out thousands and are no further forward than women who joined Match.com.

Don't make your dates dinner. If you're the coffee type, arrange to meet for a coffee. Or arrange to meet for a drink before you go on to dinner with friends. That way, there's a finite meeting time. (Believe me, some people you really don't want to be with for hours on end.) If you think you will hit it off, don't have any actual dinner plans so you can "cancel" them if all goes well.

Try hard not to judge on appearances. Many frogs have turned into princes once you look past the first layer. The factor you thought was the deal-breaker might not be. The guy who wasn't tall enough grows in stature when he turns out to be the kindest guy you've ever met.

Smile broadly even if you're dying inside because they look nothing like their photo. Who's to say you're living up to their expectations? (Sorry to be brutal, but how would you like it if his [or her] face dropped when they first saw you?)

We like people who like us. Start off with a smile and they'll be predisposed to look favorably at you.

WHAT ADVICE WOULD YOU GIVE OTHER SINGLE WOMEN WHO ARE TOO SCARED TO DATE?

Here's what women said when I asked them that question:

"Just do it! Give it a go! Nothing will shift until you shift."

"Concentrate on friendships, renew them if they've been neglected, and get out there and socialize however you like doing that. Do things you like doing for the sake of them, not necessarily to find a partner, and confidence will come, which is attractive."

"Tell your friends you're looking and they may introduce you to someone or look out for you."

"I've used eHarmony, Zoosk, Silver Singles, and Match.com. The only one I had success with is Match.com. I'm considering going back to work to meet people."

"I belong to a dating website 'appropriate' for my age group, but there are too many oldies minding their roses and talking in clichés."

"The rise of dating sites/apps has ironically contributed to the death of dating. Too much choice means guys think they're going to find someone shinier, prettier, younger on the next swipe."

"Dating apps are evil but you have to embrace them because everyone else has. It's hard to meet the right person. Use everything at your disposal."

"Whoever invented Tinder was a genius. They say it's just for sex hookups, but I've met two men through it and had two lovely relationships. It's addictive, though. I keep thinking there's someone even better and going back on there."

"My single friends and I organize get-togethers, every two months or so, for all the single people we know. We all meet up in a pub or restaurant and have a great time. Sometimes, people match up, and we've had more than a few success stories. More importantly, you make really good friends out of it."

"Get back out there but develop a thick skin. A lot of men are boring, self-obsessed, looking for younger women, or mean. Only do it when you're emotionally strong."

"Dating has changed enormously. It's much more casual now. It used to be dress up and go to dinner. Now it's 'want to meet for pizza and beer?' The pressure to put out still seems to be there though."

THE GROWN-UP'S GUIDE TO GETTING OUT THERE

Here are a few nuggets of wisdom about dating post-50, put together from personal experience, research, advice from relationship experts, and the many women who answered my questionnaires and have been there, done that. Again, they apply to everyone, regardless of sexual orientation. When I refer specifically to men, it's because the advice applies specifically to men.

Be realistic about your pulling power. Aiming for a 10 when you're a two isn't going to get you anywhere. If you're not sure how attractive you are on a scale of one to 10, ask a trusted friend, then deduct one or two points.

Get out there. Do stuff. Meet as many different people as possible. If you keep going to the same old places with the same old people and still haven't met anyone, you aren't going to. Change your habits.

Manage expectations. If you go on every date thinking they might be The One (stupid concept—who says only one person can make you happy? Are you 12?), you're going to end up mighty disappointed. Just aim to go out and have a good time. Make a few new friends.

Keep your body language open. Uncross your arms, put your hands on the table, maintain direct eye contact, smile. If you decide you like them, give them some compliments, touch their forearm, make it clear you're interested.

You're probably in charge of the date (if you're straight). Most men are crap communicators. Be curious: ask questions, find out about the person, who they really are, what they've done in their life, about their family. Steer the conversation. But don't be scared to talk about yourself. Ideally, there will be equal sharing.

Nice guys aren't boring. Don't mistake drama for love. Rollercoaster highs and lows aren't passion, they're a sign of incompatibility. Calm is good.

Aim high. The "safe bets" are just as capable of dumping you or treating you badly as riskier but more appealing partners. You might as well go for what you really want.

Don't ask for anything you can't deliver yourself. Your wish list should be things you can also offer.

The love you find will probably look nothing like what you thought it would look like. What suits you now is different than what suited you when you were younger. Be flexible. Move away from your "type" and you might just end up happier than you've ever been.

Relationships aren't everything. You don't just get love from a partner. Close friendships, family, pets, career, books, box sets, movies, travel, food, wine, solo sex—all give us pleasure. If you want one, by all means go for it. But don't turn it into your life's obsession.

Would you go out with you? If you wouldn't, sort yourself out. Take responsibility. If all your dates and relationships end badly, you're the common element. Stop blaming others for your failings.

Letting yourself be loved is as important as being able to love. Learning how to be loved is harder because it requires vulnerability.

Nothing is less attractive than desperation. It's not being desperate to admit you'd like a relationship with a particular person. It is being desperate to want a relationship so badly, you don't care who the hell it's with.

If you're not in the right mood, don't go. Showing up for a date all bitter and twisted, eyeing them with suspicion and being defensive is utterly pointless. Why bother? Stay in and watch Netflix until your mood improves, or make an appointment with a good therapist.

If you're seriously over dating, give up and make yourself happy another way. Some people have so many bad experiences they simply aren't open to any more.

Be kind to the people you date. Be gracious and respectful. The way you'd like them to treat you.

See what's really there, not what you want to see. There's positive and there's delusional. If they're over 45, they're unlikely to change now. They'll mold a little, but they're not going to change dramatically.

Stop making excuses. Adopt the "He's just not that into you" philosophy that says if he's interested, he'll be interested. Don't kid yourself.

Life's too short to waste on iffy/undecided people. If they can't decide if they want in or out at the heady beginning, they're never going to stick around when you hit the boring parts.

If they don't call or don't respond when you reach out to them, move on. Don't waste your life trying to analyze what went wrong when the answer is usually that the guy's an idiot and felt intimidated by you. Having said that . . .

Don't write people off too early. Launching into a "How dare you ignore me" rant if they don't reply to a text within a few days can come back to bite you. Things happen in people's lives that take over. Parents die. People get sick. They lose their jobs. They go on holidays. They're just not quick responders and replying within a week is actually good for them. Exit quietly and mentally write them off without letting them know you are. If they get in touch, great. If they don't, they'll think you weren't interested in them either. Win-win.

You both need to feel you're getting a good deal. It doesn't matter if one's better-looking, richer, or wittier, what matters is the balance. Ironically, it's the person who is getting the *better* deal who ends up leaving because they never feel good enough.

If you're trying really hard and it still isn't working, you're in the wrong relationship. When you find the right relationship, it's easy because you're working *with* each other. Some couples are a toxic mix: you both bring out the worst in each other.

You need three things to get you through the truly shitty times: a sense of humor, strong chemistry, and an ability to see things from each other's side.

Wait one year before trusting fully. Most people give themselves away within 12 months.

SO WHAT'S THE DEAL NOW . . .

I'M SINGLE NOW BUT FULLY INTEND ON HAVING SEX WHEN I FIND THE RIGHT PARTNER. HOW DO I KEEP MYSELF IN GOOD SHAPE SEXUALLY IN THE MEANTIME?

Masturbate regularly: it will keep your genitals fit and healthy, and your desire for sex strong. You'll find a guide on how to do that if you haven't already on page 163. There's also a guide to physically preparing your body for penetrative sex if you haven't had it for a while on page 77. Chapter 8 on sex toys also has lots of intriguing suggestions to make solo sessions fun as well as functional.

WHEN IS THE RIGHT TIME TO HAVE SEX? IS THE THREE-DATES THING STILL A THING?

Not really. The right time for you to have sex is when you want to and feel ready. It also depends on what you want from the relationship.

If you're after a fling and sex is your main motivator, why would you wait to have (safe) sex? If you think the relationship might be long-term, I'd wait for a bit. The only people who regret having sex too late didn't give clear signals they were up for it. Plenty regret having sex too early. Anyone decent isn't going to be put off by you saying you need time.

Having said that, I know loads of couples who met and slept with their partner on the same night and are still loved up years later. It's all dependent on your personal morals, personality, sexual experience, and history. Do what's right for you. There is no set time period anymore.

CAN I MAKE THE FIRST MOVE?

Damn right you can! The days of pretending we don't like sex are long gone. Whether you'll scare the horses depends on the lucky recipient's personality. If they're shy and overwhelmed by you, appearing at the door naked, wrapped in a bow, might be a bit much if you've only known them a week.

WHAT IF I ONLY WANT SEX? DO I NEED TO TELL THEM?

It depends. If it's pretty obvious you're both there for a bit of fun, spelling it out is unnecessary and a bit cringey. But if you think they're getting emotionally involved in what you thought was a friends-with-benefits thing, absolutely say something. "I'm really enjoying the sex we have but I'm not up for a relationship right now. Are you happy with that?" is all you need to say.

WHAT IF I DON'T WANT SEX AT ALL?

If you're after what your grandma would call a "companion," I'd be upfront about it quite early on. Don't think being over a certain age makes it obvious that sex won't be on offer; lots of people in their eighties are still randy little buggers. A walk in the park and cups of tea might not be all they have in mind if they invite you over for the afternoon.

The time to say you want to be celibate is either when they make an advance or they say something that suggests sex is on the agenda. If this hasn't happened within a month of seeing each other fairly regularly, bring it up regardless. Say, "I really like you and love spending time with you, but I'm not sexual anymore and not sure how important sex is for you." If you have a reason why, tell them.

Some people are happy to let sex drift into something they once did and will happily agree to a celibate but affectionate and loving relationship. Other people will exit stage left. Better to know sooner rather than later.

WHAT IF SEX NOW HURTS? DO I SAY SOMETHING BEFOREHAND OR DURING?

Say something before, during, and after. Why would you have sex that's painful and just put up with it?

It's not off-putting to admit sex hurts, it's called being human. Say, "Listen, intercourse is sometimes painful for me. I need to use lots of lube and take it slow, and you need to penetrate really slowly and stop if I tell you it hurts. Are you fine with that?" The only correct answer is "Of course!"

If the person you're sleeping with doesn't understand or looks put out, ditch them. What sort of person wants a partner to put up with pain for their own pleasure?

WHAT DO YOU THINK OF FRIENDS-WITH-BENEFITS ARRANGEMENTS?

They can be a great idea as a short-term solution—so long as neither of you has hidden motives. Trouble is, lots of people do: you're pretending it's just sex but hoping it leads to more, or they are.

Even if you leap that hurdle, if you eventually do want to find a permanent partner, friends-with-benefits arrangements take away the incentive to get out there and start looking. It's all too easy to turn up, drunk and despondent, after a date that went wrong, on their doorstep, further blurring the line between sex and love.

Some friends with benefits end up together. Most don't.

WHAT ABOUT ONE-NIGHT STANDS AND NO-STRINGS SEX?

One-night stands can be thoroughly liberating if you're in the right frame of mind and it's a positive experience. "I was traveling for business, having just finalized my divorce and trying to muster up the courage to start dating again after being with the same person for three decades. I got talking to a man in the hotel bar. Five drinks later, I told him I was terrified of getting naked with a stranger, and next thing, there I was naked! I loved it. It was just what I needed at the time," said one woman. A fling with some hot young thing might be just what you need to get over some body-image issues that your horrid ex left you with.

But if you're using casual sex to get over a still-painful split or loss, or you're feeling vulnerable and fragile, forget it. Casual sex is selfish sex—people aren't out to nurture, they're there to take. Having sex to get the cuddle at the end is never a good idea.

STRESS-FREE FIRST-TIME SEX WITH SOMEONE YOU REALLY LIKE

You'll find a guide on how to physically prepare for sex if you haven't had it in a while on page 77. But sex isn't just about being physically ready.

We all like to make out that sex isn't a big deal anymore because we live in such a sexualized society, but sex with someone you like and want to build a relationship with is a big deal. Allowing someone to see you naked—to touch, smell, and taste your body—makes you vulnerable. If you haven't got naked in front of anyone other than a long-term partner in years—maybe even decades—how is it ever not going to be a big deal? So, let's get this straight before we go any further: nerves are normal. Don't feel weird for feeling anxious. Follow your instincts and follow this guide, and all will be well.

Trust me. (Most of this is directed at man-woman pairings, simply because it's trickier for opposite-sex couples than women with women. But there are lots of things that apply to any partner combination, so please keep reading.)

Don't make a set rule of when to sleep with someone. Sometimes the first night is the right night, other times you might wait 10 dates. Another time, a few months. Let it happen organically but with one rule: you do it when you're ready, not when they're ready. Once you start having sex, you don't stop having sex. It can confuse feelings.

If you've had breast cancer and feel self-conscious, tell them. Unless you're planning on dating a teenager (I said go young, but not that young), you're dealing with a grown man. Grown men know that things like cancer happen. Teenagers are obsessed with breasts, older men not so much. They've felt more than a few; they're over it. Let him know you've had cancer and surgery and, more than likely, he'll be relieved. He can then fess up about the arthritis in his fingers and erection problems. This goes for any ailment or health issue you're worried about.

Have safe sex. Pregnancy might be unlikely but it's actually not impossible and you can still get a huge, bloody, painful blister on your vagina. Or end up with HIV. (See page 256 if you still need convincing that a condom is necessary.)

Do what makes you feel comfortable. If you want the lights out, have them out. If you want to keep some clothes on, keep them on. This also means if you've got a dodgy back or knees, feel free to position pillows for support. Warn them if there's a part of you that might make a certain position undoable.

Be prepared. Sex is less spontaneous for older women for a reason: doing it without lube is asking for painful sex and a UTI. If you feel embarrassed adding lube in front of him, go to the loo before sex to insert some high into the vagina. It will work its way down. Even if you're not planning on having intercourse, foreplay is a lot more enjoyable if you're lubricated. It also takes the pressure off worrying he won't think you're aroused if you're not lubricated.

Take baby steps. Your first few sessions might be lots of foreplay—oral sex, fingers, stroking—rather than full, penetrative sex. (You might never go for intercourse.) This is good news for both of you. We take longer to get aroused, and so do men. Not only will it give you time to get used to each other, but it also builds the tease and the erotic tension.

Remember older men need specific, firm stimulation and more of it to get and maintain an erection. If you read chapter 7, you already know how sensitive men are about any erection problems. Remember, it's unlikely he's going to get an erection just by being there with you; anticipation and simply looking at how gorgeous you are might not be enough. It's not an insult, it's called an aging penis.

Older men need firm, (preferably) experienced stimulation, even if they have taken Viagra (or similar). Don't be scared to get a grip. If you're a bit shy, take his hand and put it on his penis so he knows you're fine with him stimulating himself.

Give gentle guidance, but not too much. The first session is about connecting and being intimate together. It's not a lesson on how to give you an orgasm. If he's seriously not got a clue and you're getting nothing from it, then intervene by lifting a hand and putting it where you want it. But otherwise, be kind and encouraging. Reward things you like with obvious moans or "That feels amazing" and just don't respond as enthusiastically to things that aren't working.

Sincerity is sexy. Being genuinely aroused by someone is the biggest compliment you can give. Let them know that, even if their technique isn't perfect, you're very happy simply because it's their hand/penis/tongue touching you.

Keep it simple. Working your way through a repertoire of "tricks" looks desperate. Similarly, any slightly "out there" stuff can wait a little while. Even if you are eager to try or show off all the adventurous stuff you didn't get to try with your previous partner, hold off. Especially if he's older; older men are often far more conservative than older women. Get to know him a little first before you get the whip out.

Don't expect to orgasm. Some women find it hard not to orgasm if they've been starved of sex and finally get it. Others need to relax and trust their partner before it happens. Don't fake it, if it doesn't. If he asks, say, "I need time to get to know you before I'll relax enough for that to happen. But everything you did felt great and I'm loving lying here with you like this."

Have a sense of humor. Even if it's disastrous, if you both laugh it off, who cares? Most people muddle their way through the first time. The really good sex usually happens about four to six sessions in.

5 GOOD REASONS TO PLAY MRS. ROBINSON

It's highly probable the younger guy you choose to have sex with won't know who the hell Mrs. Robinson is. But he will know he wants you! Here's why the older woman/younger man combination works well sexually.

1. We know what we're doing. Like anything, the more experience you have, the better you are at doing something. Over the years, we've dealt with penises that won't go up, down, or do both in the same amount of time it takes to say "premature ejaculation." Younger women might have smoother thighs, but we're way more knowledgeable sexually. He can relax with us.

2. We take control. Older women aren't afraid to direct: we know our bodies well and what works and what doesn't. Plenty of young women still lie back and expect men to do all the work and refuse to guide their lovers because he should "know" what to do. Either that or they fear he'll take instruction as a criticism. Wrong. Most men love a more hands-on approach. If we want someone to touch our breasts, we take his hands and put them there.

3. We focus less on intercourse, which takes the pressure off him to perform.

4. We take our time. Because it takes us longer to warm up, we make the most of it. A slower, longer sex session is more enjoyable for both of you. He might be able to climax on cue, but a long buildup makes his orgasm better as well.

5. We let him know if we're having a good time. Why play it cool in bed? Many men name responsiveness—being able to fully arouse you—as a bigger turn-on than beauty.

Expect that you will feel vulnerable afterward. If it's the first time you've had sex since losing or splitting from a much-loved partner, you might even cry. That's OK. Just tell them how you're feeling and why. Like I said, grown-ups can handle that sort of thing.

Do make it clear being upset doesn't mean you didn't enjoy it or don't want to continue the relationship with them, though.

Even if you're screaming on the inside, "This feels like I'm cheating! This is wrong. I shouldn't have done this!" try not to panic. Be quiet, be calm, and think about that later.

The first time with someone you like can throw up all sorts of feelings. Give yourself time to sort out where you want the relationship to go later, when you've thought it through or talked to friends.

ARE YOU DYING FOR SEX? IF YOU DON'T USE A CONDOM, YOU MIGHT BE

I have one simple question for you, if you're single and sexually active: did you or are you planning to use a condom the next time you have sex with someone? If your answer is no, you're risking your health and possibly your life.

The diagnosis of STDs in the 50- to 90-year-old age group has doubled within the past 10 years. Hepatitis B and C, syphilis, HIV, chlamydia, and a drug-resistant strain of gonorrhea—with few easily recognizable symptoms—are all on the rise. Interested in contracting any of those?

The only guaranteed defense against all STDs is not to have sex at all. Herpes and warts can be spread simply by touching infected skin; pubic lice or scabies won't care if he's wearing three condoms, they'll still happily jump on the nearest strand of hair they can find.

But condoms are still a highly effective defense against most of the real nasties and will protect you against STDs spread by the exchange of bodily fluids (like semen, blood, and mucus). The riskiest behavior is having intercourse (anal or vaginal) without a condom on. If you have a sore or cut anywhere on your genitals, it's even easier for infection to spread. Remember, having oral sex can also lead to STDs. (HPV throat cancer is a very real consequence.)

Here's how to spot the person with the STD

I tricked you—you can't. Like most diseases, STDs aren't fussy and you can't pick the people who have one, often because they don't know themselves. Many STDs cause no symptoms. Having a discreet but thorough once-over of their genitals will help if they're having an attack of something at that moment—like genital warts or herpes—but it's still no predictor of what might be in their blood.

"Nice" people have STDs. The person you're already falling for may have an STD. The person who's been married for the last 30 years and only slept with one person may have an STD if their partner was unfaithful or already had an STD when they met.

If left untreated, STDs can lead to pelvic inflammatory disease and cancer of the reproductive tract in women. In men, untreated STDs can lead to cancers of the penis and anus. HPV can cause cancers of the mouth, throat, and anus in both sexes; hepatitis C puts you at risk for liver cancer.

More good news

OK, that headline's fake as well. I'm trying to frighten the hell out of you but want you to keep reading.

If you're still not convinced you're flirting with death by having unprotected sex, how about this: HIV (the virus that can lead to AIDS) is growing in the over-50 population. One study found one in six new cases of HIV diagnosed in Europe are in people over the age of 50. Twenty-seven percent of all people living with HIV/AIDS in the US are over 50.

Why? Many older people still think you can't "catch" HIV unless you share a needle for drug use or have some kind of homosexual activity. Wrong. All you need to do is have sex with that attractive person who seems awfully sweet—and not use a condom.

Real good news

Not kidding this time: most STDs are completely treatable. Even people with HIV can live long and healthy lives with antiretroviral treatment, if diagnosed early.

The problem is, most older people don't think they're at risk, so they don't ask their doctor about symptoms or risks, and lots of doctors don't discuss sexual health with older patients, assuming (wrongly in a lot of cases) that they aren't still sexually active.

If a man reports problems peeing, it's the prostate that's checked. If a woman complains of painful sex, it's assumed it's caused by vaginal dryness and a drop in hormones. STDs are rarely investigated as the culprit—but they should be.

As we get older, our immune systems weaken, making us more susceptible to infection. Viagra means many men are continuing to have penetrative sex for much longer than nature intended—and many don't use condoms or get tested. Postmenopause, thin vaginal walls, and less lubrication make the transmission of STDs and HIV even easier. If there's a minute tear or break in the skin—which there often is when you team a Viagra-hard penis with an older vagina—it's like opening the door wide and giving them a welcome drink on arrival.

Why don't older people use condoms?

Our generation tended to associate condoms with pregnancy. "Safe sex" meant not getting pregnant. Lots of older people aren't aware of how easily STDs are transmitted, have no idea what the symptoms are, have had little or no sex education, or haven't used a condom in decades and don't realize how comfortable and unobtrusive they now are. *Saga* magazine, for the over-fifties, confirms that 65 percent of people over 50 are sexually active. Lots of you are out there, dating and having sex, after divorce or the death of your partner, blissfully unaware that you need to be using condoms. Stop being naïve: sex can kill you.

It wouldn't occur to most over-fifties who've been in a long-term relationship to get a full STD checkup because it's not something they got into the habit of doing.

Use a condom. Get tested to check you haven't already been infected if you're worried. Don't have sex without a condom in a relationship until you have both been tested and given the all clear. (And until you think you can trust them to be faithful or use condoms with other people.)

If you don't want to go to your doctor, you can now buy STD and HIV self-test kits to use in the privacy of your home. Ask your pharmacist or go online; ideally, contact a sexual-health clinic, which often provides them for free, or will recommend a particular brand. The beauty of testing yourself or getting tested: you're so relieved you got the all clear, you never have sex without a condom again!

50 THINGS

YOU

ONLY KNOW

AFTER 50

MY FIFTIES ARE THE HAPPIEST time of my life. It helps that I've spent most of them in the best relationship I could possibly wish for, but it's not just about that. I feel peaceful. The fire in my belly hasn't died, but I'm happy with what I've achieved: I take on new, interesting projects but on my terms.

I worked nearly every weekend from the age of 20 to 45. I prioritized work over everything. Lucky for me, most of my friends and family were still there when I realized how ridiculous that was. I'm fitter than ever before because I've got time to both work out and calm down. Turns out yoga is transformative, not something people do when they're pretending to exercise.

I used to say shoot me if ever I say I'm content. Excitement was the goal, contentment the old fart. Now it's a glorious glass of wine and a streaming series on the sofa with my husband. I wish I could freeze time so I could stay in this decade. And I'm not the only one who reacts with "Are you kidding?" when people, always younger, say, "Wouldn't you love to be young again?"

I'm not saying I didn't enjoy the rest of my life—I've loved every precious second—but I'm loving this time the best. Probably because I finally feel like I've got a few things figured out—just like you.

You might think you know everything there is to know when you reach 18, but baby, you ain't seen nothing yet. Here are 50 things you *only* know once you're past half a century—and might want to pass on to younger women who haven't yet made it that far.

LIFE

1.   **It's not all about you.** You're not the only person and thing influencing everyone else's mood. Stop taking everything personally.

2.   **It's pointless trying to change people.** Your kids, your friends, your partner. They aren't you and don't think like you, and neither should they. Enjoy the differences rather than trying to turn everyone into mini-me.

3.   **People pleasing gets you nowhere.** Waiters who ignore you, sales clerks on their phone, people who constantly turn up late: if you don't like something, you say something.

4.   **You can't make everyone like you.** You know you're a nice person. If others don't agree, that's their issue.

5.   **Honesty isn't the best policy.** Tact, kindness, and sensitivity are. People who pride themselves on "telling it like it is" are mostly mean.

6.   **If your body is healthy, it's perfect.** Stop looking for flaws and start appreciating good health. Be happy just to have all your parts in good working order.

7.   **Being fussy isn't bad.** Time is finite. If something doesn't delight you in the first 10 minutes, ditch it for something that is worthy of your attention.

8.   **It really isn't worth sweating the small stuff.** Nothing gives you a clearer perspective than losing a friend or battling a life-threatening illness yourself.

9.   **Worrying is futile.** It never changes the outcome, and 90 percent of the time, what you fear doesn't happen.

10. **It's more important to find your tribe than be someone you aren't.** Surround yourself with people like you and no one will notice you're a little bit odd.

11. **Youth isn't wasted on the young.** Being old and content is just as enjoyable as being young and driven.

12. **Menopause is manageable.** It might fuck you up for a while, but it's a tamable beast.

13. **It's cooler to look old than desperate.** Women with faces yanked tight or pumped up like blowfish invite pity, not admiration.

14. **Be careful what you wish for.** You can never look in on other people's lives and know exactly how it feels to live them.

15. **Time waits for no man and certainly not for better circumstances.** Saying you'll do something when you meet someone/retire/find another job/move is crazy.

16. **Everyone secretly thinks they look good for their age.** But you really do.

LOVE

17. **Being alone doesn't mean you're lonely.** Nothing is lonelier than being in an unhappy relationship.

18. **You're probably not with the wrong person if you don't want to constantly have sex with your partner anymore.** Losing desire is more "natural" in long-term relationships than continuing to want sex. You'd be a freak if you wanted to slam your partner up against a wall when they walk in the door for the 15,000th time.

19. **Your partner isn't going to love you no matter what.** Saying "Harold will never cheat" is arrogant and an insult to Harold. If you love your partner, there's a reason for others to love them. Appreciate what you have while you've got it.

20. **Happy people have affairs.** Your partner's cheating on you often has nothing to do with you and your relationship, and everything to do with them.

21. **New lovers turn into old lovers.** That tempting, shiny, new person will be just as annoying in a few years as the one you've already got.

22. **Game playing gets you nowhere.** Why say you're not available to see someone you really like when you are? Swap emotional manipulation for emotional transparency.

23. **Competing with a partner makes both of you miserable.** If you're not on each other's side, what's the point?

24. **Trust your gut.** It nearly always steers you in the right direction.

25. **If you're trying really hard and it's not working,** you're in the wrong relationship.

SEX

26. **You might miss the sex you had when you were young,** but the sex you're having now isn't too bad either. It's different, that's all.

27. **It's impossible to be sexy unless you believe in yourself.** A confident lover is way more attractive than one lying there worried about cellulite.

28. **It's a relief not to be ruled by your libido.** You get yourself in a lot less trouble and staying faithful is a hell of a lot easier.

29. **Orgasms are overrated.** It really isn't about the end destination, more about having fun along the way.

30. **Enthusiasm is more attractive than a good body.** Looks fade. A genuine love of sex lasts as long as you do.

31. **There is no "right" amount of sex to have.** Who cares what everyone else is doing? Find your normal.

32. **Desire isn't the only motivator for sex.** Connection and intimacy are as important as lust. So is wanting to make your partner happy.

33. **Feeling desired is the biggest turn-on of all.** Seeing appreciation in your lover's eyes excites more than any sex trick in the book.

34. **Being selfish in bed is no bad thing.** Focus on your own pleasure, and neither has to worry if the other one is having a good time.

35. **Not getting an erection on cue is traumatic for men.** But once his penis stops being the star, sex is better. Make love with your whole body, not just your genitals.

36. **The best orgasms are often the ones you have alone.** Your vibrator won't get offended if you turn it up or down, this way or that.

37. **You don't need an erect penis to have a good time in bed.** The best, most intense partner orgasms are usually gotten through oral sex.

38. **Little blue pills aren't always the solution.** A Viagra-hard penis and a 50-plus vagina are not always a match made in heaven.

39. **It's ridiculous to feel guilty about your fantasies.** Being unfaithful in your head isn't the same as doing it in your bed.

40. **It's OK to stop having sex from time to time.** Life is stressful. Agree on a break and neither of you will freak out, thinking it's permanent.

41. **Sexuality is fluid.** Women are far more erotically plastic than men and much more likely to be aroused by the person, rather than their gender.

42. **Spontaneous sex is overrated.** Anticipation is a fine substitute.

43. **No sane woman over 50 has sex without lube.** It's as essential as toothpaste and toilet paper.

44. **The right time to have sex with someone new is when you feel ready.** That might be after "Hello," or it might be after a year.

45. **Use it or lose it.** If you don't have a partner, have sex with yourself.

46. **The female orgasm isn't inferior to his.** Give women the right stimulation and it's just as easy for us to climax.

47. **Foreplay is sex.** It's not just something you do before intercourse.

48. **Condoms aren't negotiable in new relationships.** But the person suggesting they are is.

49. **You can't have great sex if your relationship is in tatters.** Why would you want to have sex with someone you don't even like?

50. **If you're feeling bad after sex,** you're sleeping with the wrong person.

ACKNOWLEDGMENTS

I AM AN INCREDIBLY LUCKY WOMAN. This is my seventeenth book, and when I read the acknowledgments in my very first, which I wrote 20 years ago, it makes me so happy to see a lot of the same names appearing in both.

No one writes a book alone. Friends are precious; getting older makes me miss my family even more. Every time I have spare time, I mentally transport myself to their side in Australia and spend it with them. If I can't be there in the flesh, I bloody well can be in spirit. I miss them all every second of every single day. My mother, Shirley; my father, Pat, and his wife, Mo; my brother, Nigel, and his wife, Diana; my sister, Deb, and her husband, Doug; and my nephews Maddie and Charlie. You are in my heart, always.

My husband, Miles, has put up with me disappearing permanently into the office for the last six months and only interrupts to deliver icy cold glasses of wine (after 6 p.m., of course). Sorry if I boast about him in the book, but he's pretty damn adorable. So is my beautiful and bright stepdaughter, Sofia, now 18 (God help the world, she is something else).

My sister, Deb, worked with Family Planning in Australia and has an extensive knowledge of sexual health and counseling. She kindly read every chapter and gave huge encouragement, as only big sisters know how to do. My dad had been nagging me to write a sex book "for old people" long before my publishers approached me. I told him I'd love to, but that people don't buy sex books anymore. Turns out they do, Dad. (Or at least, I hope so!) My mum, still the coolest woman I have ever met, offered a fascinating perspective on sexuality and getting older. It reminded me of why all my school friends wanted her as their mum as I was growing up (and still do). My big brother, Nigel, who all my school friends wanted to run off with, kept me going with his usual witty repartee.

All my friends have done their usual job of understanding that I needed to go underground for a few months, as I always do when I write a book. I think you all know who you are by now and are bored of seeing your names in print! My agent, Vicki McIvor, is still my agent and wonderful friend—we must be into decades now, Vic! Thank you for all you do for me, both professionally and personally.

Enormous thanks, with this particular book, to Victoria Lehmann, sex therapist and lovely friend, for her expertise and eloquent interview, and to Dr. Patricia Schartau, a talented London physician who is a specialist in sexual medicine and urology, for checking all the medical bits in the book to ensure they are completely accurate. I am deeply grateful to you both.

Corinne Roberts was the publisher of my third book, *Supersex*, which was also one of the most successful. When she asked if I'd like to write about sex and midlife, I jumped at the chance to work with her again. This is my first book published with Murdoch Books, and I am already so impressed with everyone I've worked with. Enormous thanks to Lou Johnson, Jemma Crocker, Clive Kintoff, and Britta Martins-Simon for their energy, ideas, and enthusiasm. My US publisher, Chronicle Books, has been equally delightful. Cara Bedick, Mark Tauber, Jenn Jensen, and Cecilia Santini, you have all worked so hard to get the book in shape for the US market, and I am deeply grateful.

Finally, this book belongs to the many women who bared their sexual souls and gave me real and honest accounts of what it's like to be female and over 50. Thank you for trusting me with such intimate confidences. Your case histories bring the book alive.

RESOURCES

BOOKS

Anatomy of Love
Helen Fisher, PhD

Come as You Are
Emily Nagoski, PhD

The Ethical Slut
Janet W. Hardy

The Erotic Mind
Jack Morin, PhD

**A Frenchwoman's Guide
to Sex After Sixty**
Marie de Hennezel

He Comes Next
Ian Kerner, PhD

Hot Relationship
Tracey Cox

Hot Sex
Tracey Cox

**I Love You but I'm Not in
Love with You**
Andrew G. Marshall

Love Worth Making
Stephen Snyder, MD

Man Cancer Sex
Anne Katz, RN, PhD

Mating in Captivity
Esther Perel

Naked at Our Age
Joan Price

The Normal Bar
Chrisanna Northrup; Pepper
Schwartz, PhD; and James
Witte, PhD

Not Tonight Dear, I Feel Fat
Michael Alvear

Opening Up
Tristan Taormino

She Comes First
Ian Kerner, PhD

The State of Affairs
Esther Perel

Tell Me What You Want
Justin Lehmiller, PhD

**The Ultimate Guide to Sex
After 50**
Joan Price

Untrue
Wednesday Martin

What Do Women Want?
Daniel Bergner

**When You're the One
Who Cheats**
Tammy Nelson, PhD

Woman Cancer Sex
Anne Katz, RN, PhD

WEBSITES

College of Sexual and Relationship Therapists
www.cosrt.org.uk

Good in Bed
www.goodinbed.com

Healthline
www.healthline.com

Live Better With
menopause.livebetterwith.com

Lovehoney (sex-toy retailer where you'll find my Supersex and Edge product lines)
www.lovehoney.com

Mamamia
www.mamamia.com.au

Menopause Health Matters
www.menopausehealthmatters.com

MiddlesexMD
www.middlesexmd.com

Mindbodygreen
www.mindbodygreen.com

Relate (therapy and relationship support)
www.relate.org.uk

Sex & Psychology
www.lehmiller.com

Starts at 60
www.startsat60.com

PODCASTS

Mamamia: No Filter
Hosted by the brilliant and brave Mia Freedman, who has candid conversations with interesting people from all walks of life.

Quick and Dirty Tips/ Relationship Doctor
Hosted by therapist Stephen Snyder, it helps navigate the twists and turns of your love life..

TED Talks
There is an embarrassment of riches on sex, relationships, menopause, and aging here. Esther Perel's "Why Happy Couples Cheat" and "Rethinking Infidelity" are musts for anyone struggling with infidelity, on either side.

The Tracey Cox Show
You'll find my weekly radio show and podcast on Jack Radio (www.jackradio.com) and through links on my website. Everything and anything to do with sex and relationships is up for discussion, with lots of practical tips thrown in.

Where Should We Begin?
Hosted by Esther Perel. Esther counsels couples in a one-off therapy session. Heartbreaking, uplifting, informative, and fascinating, this is a rare glimpse into the intimate world of others.

REFERENCES

Here is a selection of the most interesting and relevant books, websites, and articles that I referenced for each chapter.

CHAPTER 1

Blumstein, P., and P. Schwartz. *American Couples*. New York: Pocket Books, 1983.

Godson, S. "Midlife Sex—Yes, Yes, Yes, You Must Do It!" *The Times*, June 2018. www.thetimes.co.uk/article/midlife-sex-yes-yes-yes-you-must-do-itdvt5q89t8.

Korevarr, K. "This Study on Older Adults' Sex Lives Proves Your Sex Life Isn't Doomed." *Men's Health*, July 2018. www.mh.co.za/sex-women/study-showssex-life-isnt-doomed-age-heres-exact-percentage-people-older-65-still-sex.

Nagoski, E. *Come as You Are: The Surprising New Science That Will Transform Your Sex Life*. Melbourne, Australia: Scribe, 2018.

Snyder, S. *Love Worth Making: How to Have Ridiculously Great Sex in a Long-Lasting Relationship*. New York: St. Martin's Griffin, 2018.

CHAPTER 2

Ballinger, S. E. "Psychosocial Stress and Symptoms of Menopause: A Comparative Study of Menopause Clinic Patients and Non-patients." *Maturitas* 7 (1985): 315–27.

Forever Healthy Women. https://forevher.healthywomen.org.

Gottfried, S. "How Your Hormones Really Affect Your Sex Drive + What to Do About It." mindbodygreen, 2019. www.mindbodygreen.com/0-24469/howyour-hormones-really-affect-your-sex-drive-what-to-do-about-it.html.

Hennezel, M. *A Frenchwoman's Guide to Sex After Sixty*. Vancouver, BC: Greystone Books, 2017.

Lindau, S. T., et al. "A Study of Sexuality and Health Among Older Adults in the United States." *N Eng J Med* 357 (2007): 762–74.

Oskay, U. Y., N. K. Beji, and O. Yalcin. "A Study on Urogenital Complaints of Postmenopausal Women Aged 50 and Over." *Acta Obstettcia Gynecologica Scandinavica* 84 (2005): 72–78.

Petter, O. "Nearly Three-Quarters of Women Are Uncomfortable During Sex, Study Claims." *The Independent*, February 2019. www.independent.co.uk/life-style/love-sex/painful-sex-discomfort-women-females-reasonsa8756821.html.

Portman, P. "Let's Talk About Sex, Baby: What's 'Normal' for Over-60s." *Starts at 60*, February 2019. https://startsat60.com/health/being-healthy/sex-in-older-age-what-is-normal-health-risks-what-to-expect.

Price, J. *The Ultimate Guide to Sex After 50: How to Maintain—or Regain—a Spicy, Satisfying Sex Life*. New York: Cleis Press, 2014.

Versi, E., et al. "Urogenital Prolapse and Atrophy at Menopause: A Prevalence Study." *International Urogynecology Journal and Pelvic Floor Dysfunction* 12 (2001): 107–10.

CHAPTER 3

Alvear, M. *Not Tonight Dear, I Feel Fat: How to Stop Worrying About Your Body and Have Great Sex*. Naperville, IL: Sourcebooks, 2013.

Body Logic MD. Dead Bedrooms: American Men and Women Come Clean About Their Sexless Marriages, Survey of 1,000 People. www.bodylogicmd.com/dead-bedrooms.

Nagoski, E. *Come as You Are: The Surprising New Science That Will Transform Your Sex Life*. Melbourne, Australia: Scribe, 2018.

Pells, R. "Children as Young as Three 'Worry About Being Fat or Ugly.'" *The Independent,* August 2016. www.independent.co.uk/life-style/healthand-families/health-news/children-as-young-as-three-worry-about-being-fator-ugly-a7216951.html.

Queen, Carol. *Exhibitionism for the Shy: Show Off, Dress Up and Talk Hot!* San Francisco: Down There Press, 1995.

CHAPTER 4

Hudson, R. "Feeling Stressed, Sad or Snappy." *Live Better With*, March 2019. https://menopause.livebetterwith.com/blogs/stories-info/feeling-stressed-sad-or-snappy.

National Health Service. Risks: Hormone Replacement Therapy (HRT). www.nhs.uk/conditions/hormone-replacement-therapy-hrt/risks.

Parker, J. "France: The Land That Menopause Forgot." *My Second Spring,* April 2019. https://mysecondspring.ie/blog/france-the-land-that-menopause-forgot.

Simon, J. A., et al. "Clarifying Vaginal Atrophy's Impact on Sex and Relationships (CLOSER) Survey." *Menopause* 21, no. 2 (February 2014): 137–42. www.ncbi.nlm.nih.gov/pubmed/23736862.

WebMD. Natural Alternatives to Hormone Therapy, archives. www.webmd.com/menopause/news/20000209/natural-alternatives-hormone-therapy#2.

CHAPTER 5

Flannery, J. "Taking a Closer Look at Basson's Model of the Sexual Response Cycle." Sexology International. https://sexologyinternational.com/taking-a-closer-look-at-bassons-model-of-the-sexual-response-cycle.

Morin, J. *The Erotic Mind: Unlocking the Inner Sources of Sexual Passion and Fulfillment.* New York: HarperCollins, 1995.

Perel, E. *Mating in Captivity: Unlocking Erotic Intelligence.* London: Hodder & Stoughton, 2007.

Snyder, S. "Simmering: How to Improve Your Sex Life in a Long-term Relationship." *The Times,* January 2019. www.thetimes.co.uk/article/simmering-how-toimprove-your-sex-life-in-a-long-term-relationship-ggkxvjvvc.

CHAPTER 6

Bergner, D. *What Do Women Want? Adventures in the Science of Female Desire.* New York: HarperCollins, 2013.

Boule, M. "Women Get Bored in Bed Faster Than Men." *Vice,* February 2019. www.vice.com/en_uk/article/a3bnez/women-get-bored-in-bed-faster-than-men.

Good in Bed. Good in Bed Survey, Report #1: Relationship Boredom. www.goodinbed.com/research/GIB_Survey_Report-1.pdf.

Good in Bed. Good in Bed Survey, Report #2: Sexual Adventurousness. www.goodinbed.com/research/good-in-bed-survey-report-2/index.php.

Lehmiller, J. *Tell Me What You Want: The Science of Sexual Desire and How It Can Help You Improve Your Sex Life.* London: Robinson, 2018.

Moorhead, J. "A Strong Libido and Bored by Monogamy: The Truth about Women and Sex." *The Guardian,* October 2018. www.theguardian.com/lifeandstyle/2018/oct/13/a-strong-libido-and-bored-by-monogamy-the-truthabout-women-and-sex.

CHAPTER 7

Kale, S. "Erectile Dysfunction or Performance Anxiety? The Truth Behind a Modern Malaise." *The Guardian,* October 2018. www.theguardian .com/lifeandstyle/2018/oct/18/erectile-dysfunction-performance -anxiety-truthmodern-malaise.

Kerner, I. *He Comes Next: The Thinking Woman's Guide to Pleasuring a Man*. New York: HarperCollins, 2006.

Perel, E. "Impotent Is No Way to Define a Man." *Where Should We Begin?* podcast series. www.estherperel.com/podcast.

"What Is Erectile Dysfunction?" Urology Care Foundation, June 2018. www.urologyhealth.org/urologic-conditions/erectile-dysfunction.

CHAPTER 8

Barnes, Z. "6 Lube Ingredients You Might Not Want to Put in Your Vagina." *Self,* February 2017. www.self.com/story/6-lube-ingredients-to-avoid.

Price, J. *The Ultimate Guide to Sex After 50: How to Maintain—or Regain—a Spicy, Satisfying Sex Life*. New York: Cleis Press, 2014.

Sh! Women's Erotic Emporium Ltd is another favorite in the UK. www .shwomenstore.com.

CHAPTER 9

"Are We Really in the Middle of a Global Sex Recession?" *The Guardian,* November 2018. www.theguardian.com/lifeandstyle/shortcuts/2018 /nov/14/are-we-really-in-the-middle-of-a-global-sex-recession.

Maxted, A. "'Not This Year, Darling.' The Misery of a Sexless Marriage." The *Times,* May 2016. www.thetimes.co.uk/article/hope-is-the -corrosivething-thinking-maybe-tonight-and-it-never-is-vfpxz2str.

Snyder, S. *Love Worth Making: How to Have Ridiculously Great Sex in a Long-Lasting Relationship*. New York: St. Martin's Griffin, 2018.

Watson, L. *Wanting Sex Again: How to Rediscover Your Desire and Heal a Sexless Marriage*. London: Penguin, 2012.

Weissman, Cale Guthrie. "Gen-Z Men Aren't Having Sex, and the Internet (of Course) May Be to Blame." *Fast Company,* March 29, 2019. https:// www.fastcompany.com/90327099/gen-z-men-arent-having-sex -and-the-internet-of-course-may-be-to-blame.

CHAPTER 10

Fisher, H. *Anatomy of Love: A Natural History of Mating, Marriage, and Why We Stray*. New York: Norton, 2016.

Nelson, T. "The 3 Phases of Erotic Recovery After Infidelity." Recovery, February 2015. www.recovery.org/pro/articles/the-3-phases-of -erotic-recovery-after-infidelity.

Nelson, T. *When You're the One Who Cheats: Ten Things You Need to Know.* Toronto: RL Publishing Corp., 2019.

Perel, E. "Rethinking Infidelity." TED Talk. www.youtube.com/watch?v =P2AUat93a8Q.

Perel, E. *The State of Affairs: Rethinking Infidelity.* New York: HarperCollins, 2017.

Perel, E. "Why Happy Couples Cheat." TED Talk. www.youtube.com /watch?v=JJvOTEcLapg.

CHAPTER 11

Evans, S. "Why the Over 50's Are Not Practising Safe Sex." Jo Divine. www.jodivine.com/articles/sexual-health/why-the-over-50s-are-not -practising-safe-sex.

Stepler, R. "Led by Baby Boomers, Divorce Rates Climb for America's 50 + Population." Pew Research, March 2017. www.pewresearch.org /fact-tank/2017/03/09/led-by-baby-boomers-divorce-rates-climb -for-americas-50-population.

ABOUT THE AUTHOR

Tracey Cox is one of the world's foremost writers on sex and relationships. She has been writing, researching, and talking about sex for 30 years and has toured the world as an international sex, body language, and relationship expert. Tracey has written many bestsellers, including *Hot Sex: How to Do It* and *Supersex*, and has her own product line with one of the world's most popular sex toy retailers, Lovehoney. She has a weekly column with the DailyMail.com, the world's largest English-language news website, and a weekly digital radio show, *The Tracey Cox Show*, on Jack Radio. She is married and lives in Notting Hill, London.